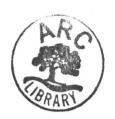

The Gestural Origin of Language

Perspectives on Deafness

Series Editors
Marc Marschark
Patricia Elizabeth Spencer

The Gestural Origin of Language

David F. Armstrong
Sherman E. Wilcox

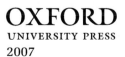

OXFORD
UNIVERSITY PRESS
2007

OXFORD
UNIVERSITY PRESS

Oxford University Press, Inc., publishes works that further
Oxford University's objective of excellence
in research, scholarship, and education.

Oxford New York
Auckland Cape Town Dar es Salaam Hong Kong Karachi
Kuala Lumpur Madrid Melbourne Mexico City Nairobi
New Delhi Shanghai Taipei Toronto

With offices in
Argentina Austria Brazil Chile Czech Republic France Greece
Guatemala Hungary Italy Japan Poland Portugal Singapore
South Korea Switzerland Thailand Turkey Ukraine Vietnam

Published by Oxford University Press, Inc.
198 Madison Avenue, New York, New York 10016

www.oup.com

Oxford is a registered trademark of Oxford University Press

Library of Congress Cataloging-in-Publication Data
Armstrong, David F.
The gestural origin of language / by David F. Armstrong
and Sherman E. Wilcox.
p. cm.—(Perspectives on deafness)
Includes bibliographical references and index.
ISBN 978-0-19-516348-3
1. Language and languages—Origin. 2. Sign language.
I. Wilcox, Sherman. II. Title.
P116.A753 2007
401—dc22   2006023748

9 8 7 6 5 4 3 2

Printed in the United States of America
on acid-free paper

This book is dedicated to the memory of

William C. Stokoe

Colleague, Mentor, Friend

Acknowledgments

Portions of this work are reprinted by permission from an article by Sherman Wilcox in *The Origins of Language: What Nonhuman Primates Can Tell Us*, edited by Barbara J. King. Copyright © 1999 by the School of American Research, Santa Fe, New Mexico.

Portions of this work are adapted from work previously published by the authors, either separately or jointly, including "Cognitive Iconicity: Conceptual Spaces, Meaning, and Gesture in Signed Languages," *Cognitive Linguistics* 15(2), pp. 119–147, © 2004 by Mouton de Gruyter, Berlin; *In the Beginning: Origins of Semiosis*, pp. 137–167, edited by M. Alac & P. Violi © 2004 by Brepols, Turnout; and "Gesture and Language: Cross-linguistic and Historical Data from Signed Languages," *Gesture* 4(1), pp. 43–75, © 2004 by John Benjamins Publishing Company, Amsterdam, and articles in the journals *Sign Language Studies* and *Behavioral and Brain Sciences* and in the *Oxford Handbook of Deaf Studies, Language, and Deafness*.

Contents

The Gestural Origin of Language

Prologue

Vision to Voice

We begin this book by inviting the reader to participate in a variation on an old thought experiment. This is an experiment that cannot and should not be conducted in the real world, but it will do no harm to speculate about its outcome. In our experiment, 24 human infants, 12 male and 12 female, are raised in a setting in which they receive food and shelter, but have no face-to-face interaction with or other communication from anyone other than their own experimental peers. There are all sorts of objects in their environment. As this is a multigenerational experiment, we assume that they figure out how to reproduce, but none of the original subjects or their descendants ever communicate with anyone from the outside world. It is widely believed that human beings have an instinctive urge to create language, so the question is this: how long, in terms of generations, does it take our subjects to create something that resembles, in complexity of lexicon and syntax, a language like English? What do their earliest attempts at communicating with each other look like? What stages do they pass through as they refine their linguistic system? Most critically from our point of view, are their first attempts to communicate with each other vocal or visible? This book represents our attempt to answer these difficult questions, and we think that most readers (even linguists if they approach this thought experiment honestly) will agree that common sense leads to the answers that we provide. This book also provides an evolutionary scenario for the emergence of human language, and we do not want to be accused of simply postulating that ontogeny recapitulates phylogeny, so we do much more than attempt to solve the puzzles proposed in this little thought experiment. However, it is worth spending a bit more time considering some answers to the questions we have posed.

With respect to our last and most critical question, we think that virtually everyone would agree that the children's first attempts to communicate in any way that might be considered referential would involve pointing to and touching or otherwise manipulating the other children and objects in their environment. Vocalization would be restricted mostly to emotional displays such as crying. We think this is a critical claim that is reinforced by the experience those of us have had who have tried to communicate with people whose language we do not know. In such circumstances, people generally resort to pointing and pantomime to make their wishes known—it occurs to very few of us to try to create, on the spot, a vocal code for use in such circumstances. It would also not occur to us to try to teach to foreigners such elements of our spoken language as would be needed to transact simple business on an ad hoc basis. Yet it is a common experience of deaf people encountering other deaf people from foreign countries to quickly negotiate a visual code that will work for at least simple communication. It was once assumed that this was possible because all deaf people used essentially the same visual, pantomimic system when they communicated with each other. It is now known, however, that the signed languages of the deaf are quite diverse and not mutually comprehensible, and just as complex grammatically as spoken languages. But it also strikes us as not surprising that deaf people find it easier to communicate with foreigners than do hearing people. Why should this be?

It is important to note that both of us have spent many years working, communicating, and, in the case of one of us, living with deaf people. We are committed to supporting and promoting the use of signed languages in the education of deaf children and as legitimate languages and forms of communication for all people. It should come as no surprise that we see these languages, or rather this form of language, as basic to the evolution of the human capacity for language in general, and it is our aim to show what recent evidence from the study of human signing and gesture has to tell us about the history of this most essential of human abilities.

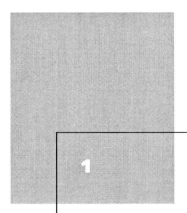

1

Grasping Language

Sign and the Evolution of Language

1 Gestural Theories of the Origin of Language

Speculation about how languages originate and evolve has had an important place in the history of ideas, and it has been intimately linked to questions about the nature of the signed languages of the deaf and human gestural behavior in general. It can be argued that, from a phylogenetic perspective, the origin of human sign languages is coincident with the origin of human languages; sign languages, that is, are likely to have been the first true languages. This is not a new perspective—it is perhaps as old as nonreligious speculation about the way human language may have begun. For example, in Plato's *Cratylus*, Socrates speculates about the nature of the sign language used by the deaf in relation to the origin of words (Jowett, 1901: 662):

SOCRATES: [H]ow do the primary names which precede analysis show the natures of things, as far as they can be shown; which they must do, if they are to be real names? ... Suppose that we had no voice or tongue, and wanted to communicate with one another, should we not, like the deaf and dumb, make signs with the hands and head and the rest of the body?

HERMOGENES: There would be no choice, Socrates.

SOCRATES: We should imitate the nature of the thing; the elevation of our hands to heaven would mean lightness and upwardness; heaviness and downwardness would be expressed by letting them drop to the ground; the running of a horse, or any other animal, would be expressed by the most nearly similar gestures of our own frame.

Here is expressed clearly the idea that gesture is somehow "natural"—we might say iconic—that there is a more direct connection between visible gestures and the things they refer to than is true of spoken words and things in the world. We also see in this Platonic dialogue the idea that the arbitrariness and abstractness of speech is necessary for the full development of human thought, an idea that will also continue to crop up.

During the French Enlightenment of the eighteenth century, philosophers such as Condillac speculated that sign languages may have preceded speech (see Hewes, 1996). Some of these writers were aware of the work of teachers of the deaf such as Pereire, and there appears to have been feedback between the *philosophes* and the Abbé de l'Epée, who opened the first school for the deaf in France in the late eighteenth century, as the theories of deaf education and the origin of language evolved in tandem (Lang, 2003; Rosenfeld, 2001).

In his day, Epée was widely credited with inventing the sign language used by French deaf people. What now appears likely is that there were already varieties of signed language in use by the deaf people of the various regions in France at the time he opened his school and that he systematized the use of these signs for the purpose of teaching deaf pupils to read and write the French language, through a system that came to be known as Methodical Signs. This system was probably modeled on French syntax to some extent and certainly involved fingerspelling of French words. This sort of appropriation of the signs from the natural sign languages of the deaf for use in a language system modeled on the local spoken language has also occurred repeatedly in deaf education. We will be exploring how these natural sign languages differ in structure from spoken languages and invented educational signing.

The publication in 1859 of Darwin's *Origin of Species* heightened interest in the origin of human beings and their languages. Darwin set the stage for future theorists by stating at the close of his great book that "much light will be thrown on the origin of man and his history." Following publication of the *Origin*, a period of speculation commenced about how languages may have arisen in the course of human evolution. This statement by Edward Tylor (1865; quoted in Kendon, 2002: 38–39) is perhaps representative of the better thought-out theorizing of the time:

The Gesture-language and Picture writing, insignificant as they are in practice in comparison with Speech and Phonetic writing, have this great claim to consideration, that we can really understand them as thoroughly as perhaps we can understand anything, and by studying them we can realize to ourselves in some measure a condition of the human mind which underlies anything which has as yet been traced in even the lowest dialects of Language, if taken as a whole. Though, with the exception of words in which we can trace the effects either of direct emotion, as in interjections, or of imitative formation, as in 'peewit' or 'cuckoo,' we cannot at present tell by what steps man came to express himself in words, we can at least see how he still does come to express himself by signs and pictures, and so get some idea of this great movement, which no lower animal is known to have made or shown the least sign of making.

We very much support this idea—that by examining what is known about the invention of visual varieties of language, especially the signed languages of the deaf but also writing—we can learn much about the way language in general probably emerges.

However, much of the speculation at this time was undisciplined and unsupported by evidence, such that, in 1866, the Linguistic Society of Paris banned discussion of the topic at its meetings (Hewes, 1996). Thus article 2 of the bylaws of the Linguistic Society of Paris, adopted March 8, 1866: "The Society will accept no communication concerning either the origin of language or the creation of a universal language."

The London Philological Society followed suit in 1872 (Kendon, 2002: 42). It is interesting that the Paris Society chose to associate speculation about the origins of language with attempts to create a universal language, as there has also long been an association between signed languages and the idea that there must be some "universal" form of signing that could be understood by all deaf people, or even all people regardless of their nationality. Again, this has probably emerged as a result of the notion that signing is somehow characteristically iconic and therefore "natural." The truth, of course, is that the signed languages of deaf people vary, just as do the spoken languages of hearing people, and they are just as mutually unintelligible. However, it is a common observation that deaf people from different language communities find it easier to develop a mutually intelligible gestural code than do hearing people from divergent speech communities. This probably has to do to some extent with the underlying iconicity of all signed languages, as well as the experience built up by deaf people through lifetimes of having to find ways of communicating with hearing people who are ignorant of sign languages.

By this time, that is, the late nineteenth century, the idea that signed languages like those used by deaf people might have something to do with the origin of language in general had become quite pervasive in the thinking even of nonscholars. Amos Kendall was a significant political figure in the city of Washington during the mid-nineteenth century, and he was a confidant of Andrew Jackson. He was also responsible for starting a school for deaf and blind children in the U.S. capital and for hiring Edward Miner Gallaudet to run it. The school evolved into the present—day Gallaudet University. This passage is from Kendall's speech at the inauguration of the College for the Deaf and Dumb (later Gallaudet University) in 1864 (Gallaudet, 1983: 211):

> If the whole human family were destitute of the sense of hearing, they would yet be able to interchange ideas by signs. Indeed, the language of signs undoubtedly accompanied if it did not precede the language of sounds. . . . We read that Adam named the beasts and birds. But how could he give them names without first pointing them out by other means? How could a particular name be fixed upon a particular animal among so many species without some sign indicating to what animal it should thereafter be applied? . . . If a company of uneducated deaf-mutes were, for the first time, brought into contact with an elephant, without knowing its name, they would soon devise a sign by which he should be represented among themselves. So, were it possible for a company of adults with their senses entire to be placed in a similar situation, they would probably point him out by a sign accompanied by some exclamation, and the exclamation might become the name of the animal. Thenceforward the perfect man would convey the idea of an elephant by sound, while the deaf-mute could only do it by a sign.

Except for the presence of Adam in this account, and the use of politically incorrect terms to denote deaf and hearing people, some of its elements are not too different from those of contemporary gestural scenarios for the origin of language.

This sort of speculation might at first seem somewhat paradoxical. Most human languages, of course, are spoken. Speech is the dominant form of human communication. What could be gained theoretically by assuming a period in human history in which visual-gestural communication was predominant? The scenario presented in Kendall's speech addresses some of the key points, the most basic being how to get from an object or an event in the material world to an apparently arbitrary vocal symbol. The idea of primitive humans making mimetic gestures to refer to objects and events in their environment and coupling these with vocalizations may seem simple-minded, but it also has explanatory appeal. Hewes (1976: 486) points out that even following the bans on publication of such theorizing by major scholarly societies, speculation about the gestural origin of language continued into the 1880s. Nevertheless, for most of the century following the Paris Society's ban on its discussion, serious scholars assiduously avoided the topic of language origins, although there were exceptions, such as the German psychologist Wilhelm Wundt (487).

One could ask if this might not have been a good thing. After all, what can we ever know with certainty about how our ancient ancestors communicated? Behavior, famously and axiomatically, does not fossilize, and communication events are the most ephemeral of behaviors, but questions about the evolution of our ability to create languages are central to our understanding of our nature and our origins, questions about which human beings are intensely curious. In any event, in the early 1970s, a concerted movement to reopen the topic to serious scholarly study began to emerge in the United States. Important evidence was accumulating in a variety of fields that could be brought to bear on this question, most significantly, from our point of view, research pioneered by William C. Stokoe that suggested that full-fledged languages could exist in the visual-gestural mode.

It is also significant that the Paris Linguistic Society's ban on discussion of language origins, which helped to take discussion of the role of sign and gesture in this process off the table, was followed in 1880 by the infamous international conference in Milan of educators of the deaf. The attendees of this conference took a position in favor of oral-only education for the deaf and against the use of signed languages in schools for the deaf. During a Victorian era that was steeped in notions of progress, a move toward oral-only education for the deaf, to the exclusion of any use of sign language, had broadly taken hold. The usual statement of the goal of oral education for the deaf was that it was designed to "return the deaf to society." Baynton (2002) describes the chilling effect that the rise of oralism had not only on the *use* of signed languages in the education of the deaf, but on the *study* of signed languages as well, study that had flourished prior to 1880. Interest in the scientific study of sign languages had reached its nadir during the first half of the twentieth century, as had interest in gestural theories of language origins, prior to Stokoe's initial work.

Baynton (2002) asks not only why oralism rose to prominence but why sign languages themselves were devalued at this time. He concludes that the early theories of language evolution that included an initial signing or gestural stage are part of the answer. A sort of linguistic "Darwinism" arose, according to which earlier forms were replaced by more "fit" or "adaptive" forms; thus, perhaps, sign was replaced by speech because speech was inherently superior.

That the signed languages of the deaf were not of interest to mainstream structural linguists of the first part of the twentieth century is made abundantly clear in Edward Sapir's classic book *Language: An Introduction to the Study of Speech* (1921: 21):

> Still another interesting group of transfers are the different
> gesture languages, developed for the use of deaf-mutes, of
> Trappist monks vowed to perpetual silence, or of communicat-
> ing parties that are within seeing distance of each other but are
> out of earshot. Some of these systems are one-to-one equiva-
> lences of the normal system of speech; others, like military
> gesture-symbolism or the gesture language of the Plains Indians
> of North America (understood by tribes of mutually unintelli-
> gible forms of speech) are imperfect transfers, limiting them-
> selves to the rendering of such grosser speech elements as are
> an imperative minimum under difficult circumstances.

This statement is particularly interesting because it represents two prejudices that were shown to be wrong by Stokoe (1960) and subsequently by many others: language is spoken (note that according to his title, Sapir's book about language is really about the study of speech), and the signing done by deaf people is simply a substitution code for speech (if it is even that sophisticated).

Theorists such as us, who are about to propose a gestural origin theory, need to be aware that invidious claims about the inferiority of the signed languages of the deaf have been based to some extent on the gestural ori-gin theories of a previous generation and the offhand dismissals of earlier linguists like Sapir. We, are, therefore, explicit about the fact that the natural sign languages used by modern deaf people are fully modern languages in every meaningful sense. We will argue, however, that aspects of the struc-tures of these languages and the historical processes through which these languages came into existence can shed light on the way human language in general most probably evolved.

2 Sign Language, Gesture, and Language Origins

Stokoe initiated the modern scientific study of signed languages by draw-ing on the insights of anthropological and structural linguists who had come to realize that all languages have regular structures at a level below that of the individual word. According to the terminology of linguistics, they have sublexical or phonological structure. This structure is based on systems of contrast—differences in meaning must be based on perceptible differences in language sounds, as in *bat* and *hat*. It is this sublexical structure that makes phonetic writing possible, and all spoken languages have it. Stokoe's contribution was to show that what came to be called American Sign Language (ASL) has such a structure and that it, too, can be written in a phonetic-like script (Stokoe, 1960; Stokoe, Casterline & Croneberg, 1965). By devising a workable script, he was able to convince other language scholars that ASL employs such a system of linguistic contrast, that it has a regular internal structure, and that it is, therefore, not simply ad hoc pantomime or a corrupt visual code for English.

During the early 1970s, Stokoe began to see that his work on ASL might have a larger significance, beyond the development of increasingly complex linguistic studies and the support these were providing for the reform of deaf education. At this time, Stokoe became interested in the newly reinvigorated scientific study of the origin and evolution of the human capacity for language. Stokoe joined a small group of scholars, including Gordon Hewes (1973), who began to synthesize new information from paleontology, primatology, neuroscience, linguistics, and sign language studies into more coherent scenarios for the evolution of language (see Harnad, Steklis, & Lancaster, 1976). During the past quarter century, these scenarios have grown more sophisticated and plausible, due in large part to Stokoe's efforts.

Stokoe concerned himself especially with evolutionary problems that might be solved by postulating a signing stage in human evolution. He participated in several important symposia on this topic, one of which resulted in the book *Language Origins* (Wescott, 1974). Stokoe came to believe that iconic manual gesture must have played a key role in the transition from nonhuman primate communication to human language. In making this assertion, he was rediscovering a line of thinking that went back at least to the Abbé de Condillac, and it can be traced through the quotation earlier from Amos Kendall. According to this line of thinking, the introduction of iconic manual gesture might solve the problem of attribution of meaning to arbitrary vocal signals—iconic gestures that resemble the things they refer to might form a bridge to the symbolic relationship of speech sounds to their referents.

But Stokoe went a step beyond this to suggest that iconic manual gestures might also have been involved in the thornier question of how grammar originated. He put it in these terms in 1976 at the seminal conference on the origin and evolution of language organized by the New York Academy of Sciences (see Harnad, Steklis, & Lancaster, 1976):

> Transitive verb signs in contemporary, highly encoded sign
> languages may be interesting linguistic fossils, if, like rocks put
> to modern uses, they contain traces of ancient processes.
> Grasping an object, as an action or observed event, presents
> both a verbal and a nominal appearance. When a hand holding
> nothing re-presents in mimicry its own real action of grasping,

> the gSign [gestural sign] immediately produced (for any
> observer including the maker who perceives a resemblance)
> still works in contemporary sign languages either as a verb or as
> a verb plus inanimate noun—the absent or displaced object. It
> seems likely that the latter use, of sign for the whole event,
> antedates the former, which shows the verb part abstracted
> from the, at first undivided but in fact divisible, gSign signal.
> (Stokoe, 1976: 509)

This description of an iconic manual sign as having at the same time
the potential value of a word or a sentence goes to the question at the heart
of Chomskyan linguistics, which posits syntax as the defining characteristic of human languages—how do languages come to refer not only to
objects and events but also to the infinite number of possible relationships
among them?

As we will see later, Stokoe went on to elaborate on this idea in an
article entitled "Semantic Phonology" (1991). We can get the flavor of his
more extended argument in this brief quotation from the article describing his analysis of an iconic manual sign into protogrammatical elements:

> An s-p [semantic-phonological] noun-verb unit represents a
> word of sign language, it is both an agent-verb construct and in
> the lexicon a formal noun or verb or other part of speech of the
> language, and it can combine in the normal way with others
> like it to make a grammatical noun-verb structure. This struc-
> ture in turn has meaning (actually it always had). (112)

Armstrong, Stokoe, and Wilcox developed this idea further in the book
Gesture and the Nature of Language in 1995. In order to illustrate the idea
that what appears to be a single iconic manual gesture might also have the
structure of a prototypical sentence, Armstrong, Stokoe, and Wilcox (1995:
22) describe the production of the ASL sign meaning "capture" or "grasp,"
contrasting it with the sign for "know," which involves touching the bent
hand to the forehead:

> This time the hand begins less bent or fully open; the flexion at
> the elbow is less; and the upper arm instead of extending
> rotates at the shoulder joint to bring the forearm and hand
> across in front of the body until the moving hand closes around
> the upright forefinger of the other hand. This too might be
> called a motivated sign. As just described, it means 'catch'; its
> iconicity is even more obvious than in the sign for 'know.' The
> active hand caught or grasped the finger of the other hand . . .
> The iconicity now is not between a sign and a single thing or

action it signifies but between the whole gestalt of something acting, its action, and the result, the patient it acts upon. In other words, this manual-brachial gesture meaning 'grasp' or 'catch' is also a complete transitive sentence: It has a subject, a verb, and a direct object, or, in semantic terms, an agent, action, and patient.

One of the purposes of this book will be to show how this idea can be extended beyond speculation about the origin of language into the realm of historical linguistics and the processes of grammaticalization, the processes by which grammatical structures emerge from the lexicon of a language.

3 Vision versus Audition

The differences between the two major human senses and the neurological and cognitive systems that support them may seem obvious to most people, but it is necessary to be explicit if we are to support the current argument that true human language began in the visual medium. We begin by considering the importance of what appears to be a uniquely well developed human neurological attribute—cross-modal association, the ability to freely combine sensory input from more than one modality, that is, vision, hearing, and somatosensory input into higher order concepts and images. In the realm of language and cognition in general, it could be argued that a primary function of metaphor and other figurative spoken language is to enable the translation of essentially visual information into the abstraction that sound is to us. Not surprisingly, the only other mammal that seems to have this ability developed to anything like its extent in humans may be the chimpanzee. In fact, it may be that it is a highly developed ability to do cross-modal association that allows us to construct and use the symbols of language (Laughlin & D'Aquili, 1974: 52). Cross-modal transfer of sensory information is associated with the cortex of the inferior parietal lobe and surrounding regions, an area of the brain that has grown dramatically during the course of human evolution. This functional region is also sometimes referred to as the parietal/occipital/temporal area (POT). But why would this sort of sensory integration be so important to the appearance of human language?

One of the many curious things about language is that for most people it is not expressed and perceived in the dominant human sensory modality, which, unquestionably, is vision. Human beings are primates, and because they are primates, when they gather information about the world, they gather it primarily through their eyes. Primates are so visually oriented presumably because their ancestors' primary adaptation was arboreal, that is to life in trees. As we have noted elsewhere (Armstrong, Stokoe, & Wilcox, 1995: 48) there is a very simple, very draconian Darwinian explanation for the primacy of the sense of vision in primates—a leaping monkey that misses its grip is likely to be a dead monkey. This mode of life, especially when it involves feeding on small food items like insects and fruits, also requires a great deal of manual dexterity and eye-hand coordination, all of which are hallmarks of the primate adaptation. Because light is relatively unaffected by passage through air, and except possibly for *echolocation* (described later), vision is the only way to collect completely reliable information about the precise sizes, shapes, and locations of objects at a distance. The possession of exceptional acuity and binocularity for depth perception is, thus, fundamental to the adaptation of arboreal creatures such as primates.

Because we are so visually oriented, it is hard for us to imagine the sensory capabilities of some other animals. When we want to know the truth about a crime, we *look* for an *eyewitness* who *saw* it done. We tend not to accept *hearsay*. *Seeing*, after all, is believing. But if we were carnivores and not primates, we would probably want to sniff out a nosewitness. Just as we cannot *picture* how a dog constructs its olfactory world, we find it similarly hard to *visualize* the way a bat or a dolphin is able to detect the shapes of distant objects using its auditory sense, through a process called *echolocation*. In this case, the sounds perceived by the animal were also created by the animal, but this extraordinary sensory feat is carried out completely in the auditory medium. The information—carrying capacity of the auditory sense in humans and other primates is much more limited. Humans can certainly make some judgments about the type of an object or animal and its approximate location by the sounds that it makes, but to understand the difference between the human senses of sight and hearing, we need only contrast the relative ease of mobility of deaf people and blind people. Who is more at risk walking near a cliff on a still day, a deaf person or a blind person?

If our sense of hearing is so inferior as an information-gathering device, why do we use it to support what is undeniably our most important communication and information—gathering system—language? Before we move to a consideration of possible reasons for this, we again want to reinforce the idea that one of the cognitive functions that may make this possible is cross-modal sensory association or transfer in humans and the evolution, in terms of size and complexity, of the brain structures that enable it. This sort of association in nonhuman primates tends to imply the need for reinforcement to make the link; that is, it implies a lack of voluntary control. It is worth mentioning here that there have been claims for the relatively early appearance of a well—defined, human-like inferior parietal lobe in the human fossil record (see Corballis, 2002: 149 for a discussion of this evidence).

If Laughlin and D'Aquili are correct, the ability to abstract out a mental construct that involves a variety of sensory input is what allows human beings to attach arbitrary or conventional signs to these concepts. But we will argue throughout this book that these signs must first be grounded or embodied as a result of direct analogy to the world around us, and that this must first occur in the visual modality before it can be transferred to the auditory. Later in this book, we will also discuss possible reasons for a shift in the major language—carrying channel in humans from vision to audition, but there can be no doubt in this regard that visible gesture never left the scene—it continues to be essential in the face—to—face communication of all people, hearing as well as deaf. It can, in fact, be quite difficult for people conversing by telephone to voluntarily suppress the manual gestures that normally accompany their speech.

4 This Book

Our argument begins with an exploration of the current evidence for the participation of gesture in the origin and evolution of the human capacity for language. The particular grasping gesture that we described earlier has a central metaphorical role in this argument. There is powerful new evidence from neurology that gestures such as the grasping gesture are underlain by groups of neurons that have been dubbed "mirror neurons" by their discoverer (Rizzolatti & Arbib, 1998). Mirror neurons have been identified in monkeys and human beings, and in some monkeys they are found in areas of the frontal cortex that may be homologous with Broca's area in humans. Mirror neurons appear to be active when a particular manual activity is being either performed or perceived by a primate, and it is significant that they appear to be tuned to specific kinds of manual activities such as grasping. Rizzolatti and Arbib (1998) have hypothesized that mirror neurons represent the neural substrate for communication by gesture, because of the power of this manual activity to elicit in the observer the same neurological state as exists in the sender—opening the way perhaps for comprehension of a manual gesture by its observer. Corballis (2002), among others, has, as we will see later, developed a comprehensive theory deriving language from mirror neuron–mediated gesture, and, in particular, showing how the brain laterality associated with language and handedness in humans may have emerged through an evolutionary process involving such manual gestures.

In addition, in chapter 2, we will be concerned also with the evolution of various anatomical features of modern humans that appear to facilitate the development and use of language, including those features that enable upright bipedalism and significant changes in the upper respiratory tract, as well as aspects of the brain, including Broca's and Wernicke's areas of the lateralized cerebral cortex. The fossil evidence suggests that the earliest hominids were likely to have had more facility for communication through visible gesture than for communication involving complex vocalization. We will also examine the evidence concerning the gestural and other language-like behavior of nonhuman primates, especially the behavior of the closest living relatives of modern humans, the great apes of Africa.

Next, in chapter 3, we review the literature from researchers such as David McNeill, Adam Kendon, and others that reveals psychological and linguistic evidence for deep connections between gesture and speech. We relate this information to the question of the origin of grammar, through consideration of the iconic structures in signed languages that have been called "classifier constructions." We also consider the relative demands on brain development that result from sign and speech, and we trace the processes of grammar development in the historical development of signed languages.

In "Talk Is Cheap: Sarcasm, Alienation and the Evolution of Language," John Haiman noted that "with insignificant exceptions like 'ouch' and 'boo hoo,' we cannot observe how words developed out of nonwords; however far back we go, it seems that all of our etymologies of words trace to nothing but other older words" (1998b: 00). It is interesting that this problem was recognized by Socrates in Plato's *Cratylus*. A central problem for the evolution of language is not merely the emergence of words but also grammar. A popular claim is that the grammars of all languages are a reflection of the single genetically programmed universal grammar that emerged only once, among the ancestors of modern humans. Yet linguists such as Haiman, Joan Bybeee, Elizabeth Traugott, and Paul Hopper have shown that grammar continually develops out of nongrammar.

In chapter 4, we present evidence from several signed languages for the emergence of grammar from the words (signs) of these languages. We go even further, however, and document how signed words, in fact, develop out of nonwords—out of gesture by the same fundamental processes. This is the advantage that the study of signed languages uniquely offers— we can observe as new languages actually emerge, as, for example, in the case of Nicaraguan Sign Language (NSL). Here we connect the emergence of language to a process long studied in the evolution of animal behavior generally—the process of ritualization.

In chapter 5, we consider evidence for the ubiquity of iconicity in signed languages, a consequence we believe of their transmission in the visual medium. Adopting a cognitive grammar framework (Langacker, 1987, 1991a, b), we describe the iconic representation of space and time in signed languages. Iconicity is understood not as a relation between language and external reality, but as a mapping within multidimensional conceptual space, between the semantic and phonological poles of a symbol—again, we encounter what Stokoe called semantic phonology, as we described it earlier. This mapping can vary in distance from one of identity or self-symbolization, in which the thing represents itself, to one of iconicity, in which the semantic and phonological poles reside in roughly the same conceptual space. At further distances in conceptual space, the semantic and phonological poles become so unrelated that we arrive at what linguists call the arbitrariness of the sign, where the relationship appears to be one of convention only. The conceptual spaces of most interest here are those that are "embodied," that map onto the bodies of individuals as they interact in the construction of discourse.

In chapter 6, we propose a reunification of language and gesture. We claim that only by starting with the premise that signed languages are the original and prototypical languages can we achieve a unity of speech and sign as forms of language.

Rather than searching for this unity in ever more abstraction away from the linguistic material itself, the gestural substance of linguistic communication, we claim that unity can be achieved by seeing language as grounded in embodied action—visible movement.

Chapter 7 provides direct evidence for the theory that language emerges first visually and gesturally by examining the only archeological and historical evidence that bears directly on this issue: archeological evidence for the invention of writing and historical evidence concerning the emergence of the signed languages of the deaf. We will show that the development of these linguistic systems has followed similar paths at places and at times that were widely separated, so that these events can be considered to be independent of one another and, thus, reflective of some fundamental human attribute.

Finally, we propose that the evolutionary processes that led to the emergence of language in our species can be unified with those that lead to the ongoing emergence of linguistic forms through ritualization of gestural behavior. Our central thesis is that the study of signed languages opens a window on this process that is not available through the study of speech.

TWO

Language in the Wild

Paleontological and Primatological Evidence for Gestural Origins

1 The Nature of the Fossil Evidence

Debate continues to rage among practitioners of the sciences of language concerning the positing of mental devices as a goal of the enterprise. According to Jackendoff (2002), mentalism should continue to be a guiding principle of linguistic science and the elucidation of mental structures one of the goals of evolutionary study (a point that is reinforced by Hauser, Chomsky, & Fitch, 2002). Whatever the status of hypothesized mental structures in modern humans, we do not believe that pursuing them in human ancestors is likely to be profitable. The only evidence we have concerning the linguistic and communication abilities of the first hominids is indirect and must be inferred from the fossil evidence. Even the anatomical evidence concerning the nature of the population of animals that diverged in the direction of modern humans on the one hand and modern chimpanzees on the other is very sketchy at best. Therefore, the best approach to speculating about the capabilities of these creatures is to triangulate from evidence concerning the communication abilities of modern chimps and gorillas, modern humans, and the fossil evidence concerning the anatomical and neurological features of the common ancestor and early hominids. In the first chapter, we introduced some of the evidence for the anatomical features of the common ancestor. Here we will elaborate on that evidence briefly, and then go into a more detailed discussion of what is known about the linguistic or language-like behavior of modern great apes, especially chimpanzees (including bonobos) and gorillas.

Several lines of evidence converge to support the idea that gesture-based language might have preceded speech in human phylogeny: (1) paleontological evidence for human anatomical evolution; (2) primatological evidence concerning the behavior of the closest living relatives of human beings; and (3) neurological evidence concerning the organization of the substrates for linguistic behavior in the brain.

It is necessary first to review what is known about the evolutionary relationships of human beings and our closest living relatives, the apes of Africa: bonobos (sometimes referred to as pygmy chimpanzees), chimpanzees, and gorillas. Bonobos and chimpanzees are both members of the genus *Pan,* and hereafter both species will be referred to collectively as chimpanzees. Comparative studies of DNA have shown that humans are extremely closely related to the African apes, but that they are probably more closely related to chimpanzees than to gorillas (for an accessible discussion of this evidence, see Fouts & Mills, 1997: 52–58). Human beings in turn all belong to the genus *Homo,* which has only one living species, *Homo sapiens.* The traditional taxonomic term for the human lineage after its separation from the lineage that led to modern chimpanzees is the primate family Hominidae, the hominids. Traditional classifications of the African apes group them with the great apes of Asia, orangutans, in a family called the Pongidae. The Hominidae and Pongidae, in turn, were grouped together in a superfamily, the Hominoidea. Recent genetic studies have shown clearly that gorillas and chimpanzees are more closely related to humans than they are to orangutans, so having a taxon, the Pongidae, that includes all of the apes but not humans would seem to violate the spirit of a hierarchical classification system based on evolutionary relationships. Although there has been a recent move among primate taxonomists to recognize the closeness of the relationships among humans, chimps, and gorillas by including all of these primates in the hominids, we will follow the traditional use of this term and use it to refer only to human beings and their extinct relatives following the split with the ancestor of chimpanzees.

There is evidence that the human lineage separated from the line leading to modern chimpanzees 6 to 7 million years ago and that the common ancestor may have resembled modern chimpanzees in terms of locomotor and postural adaptations and brain size (see Armstrong, 1999: 21–30; Begun, 1994; Richmond & Strait, 2000). The anatomical features of chimpanzees and gorillas that are of greatest interest here, given the very close genetic relationship between these apes and humans, are those relating to locomotion and brain size and structure, assuming as we suggested earlier that the common ancestor of humans and chimpanzees resembled a modern chimpanzee.

It is significant that chimpanzees and gorillas share a unique form of locomotion, one that is as unusual as the upright, striding, bipedal gait of modern humans. Chimpanzees and gorillas are knucklewalkers, and, occasionally, brachiators, although adult gorillas are very large and heavy and do not spend much time in trees. What this means is that the African apes share a set of anatomical peculiarities, including hands with elongated fingers and shortened thumbs, arms that are relatively long relative to trunk length and legs that are relatively short, and what Napier (Napier & Napier, 1967) has called a "facultative bipedalism." In other words, because their arms are long and their legs short, their habitual posture when walking is relatively upright. When hanging from tree limbs in the typical brachiator mode, their posture is also relatively upright. Evidence supporting the idea that the common ancestor of humans and apes was a knucklewalker has recently been compiled by Richmond and Strait (2000).

It has been hypothesized that the adoption of upright bipedalism characteristic of the hominids is the solution to the relatively inefficient knucklewalking of the apes in more open environments. With respect to the evolution of language, we argue that this change in posture was fundamentally important, because it freed the hands for gesturing and it placed the trunk in full view of conspecifics with which a hominid wished to communicate. The body could now be used as the platform upon which to make gestural signs, and a developing capacity for language was, thus, embodied from the very beginning of its history.

This is not to devalue the importance of the face in primate communication—it continues to play an important role in the gestural communication of monkeys, apes, and humans, but the freeing of the hands and upper body for full participation in gestural communication was surely a giant step along the road to real language. It is also worth mentioning the face, because it has been shown during the recent expansion of research on sign language that facial gestures play a critical role in the grammars of signed languages. There is recent evidence of a fundamental linkage between facial expression, posture, and vocal calls in the communication of rhesus monkeys (Ghazanfar & Logothetis, 2003), such that these monkeys "sometimes accompany their vocalizations with distinctive body postures and facial expressions." We will later be describing linkages between manual gesture and speech in human communication, but it is clear that communication by vocalization cum gesture has a very long history in the primate order.

There are two well-established genera of hominids: *Australopithecus*, whose members are extinct, some of them probably ancestral to modern humans, and *Homo*, which includes several well-established extinct species, such as *Homo erectus*, in addition to *Homo sapiens*. Several other genera have been proposed for fossils older than about 3 million years, including *Ardipithecus,* but the fossil evidence for hominids preceding the australopithecines is still relatively limited (for a readable account of the many controversies surrounding the recent discoveries of hominid fossils in the range of 4 to 7 million years old, see Gibbons, 2006). All of this evidence, including that for the australopithecines, is from Africa. The earliest hominid known to have lived outside of Africa belongs to the species generally known as *Homo erectus*, which is now known to have been distributed widely throughout the Old World (fig. 2.1).

During the past several decades, paleoanthropologists have established that bipedalism is the defining anatomical trait of the hominid lineage—it emerged before the enlargement of the brain, the other striking peculiarity of human anatomy (for a recent summary of the evidence, see Tattersall, 1999). What is most significant here is that by roughly 3 million years ago, the time of the famous *australopithecine* Lucy, bipedalism was firmly established and the human hand had begun to move toward its modern configuration (Marzke, 1996). What is equally clear is that the brain had not yet begun to enlarge. Students of language evolution have considered the shape of the skull, especially its base (basicranium), important because they take it as indicative of whether or not the larynx has descended from the relatively high position characteristic of most mammals and nonhuman primates to the relatively low position characteristic of adult humans. This

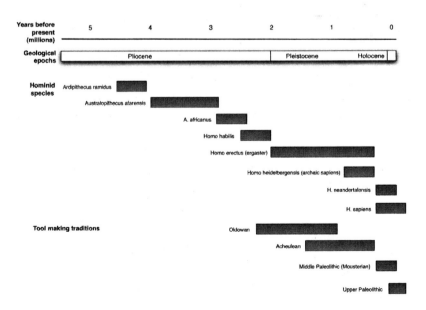

Figure 2.1. Hominid timeline.

low position of the larynx allows for an expansion of the pharynx and the production of a wider range of vowel sounds. Because the vocal apparatus is essentially made of soft tissue, it does not fossilize, and the position of the larynx has to be inferred from the shape of the basicranium—the more it is bent or flexed, the lower the larynx can be assumed to be. In nonhuman primates, the base of the skull is relatively flat, and in modern humans it is relatively flexed.

In fact, it has been argued that hominids as recent as members of *Homo erectus*, less than 2 million years ago, would have been incapable of making the full range of modern speech sounds (Lieberman, 1991: 74–76; and see Walker & Shipman, 1996). This argument has been based on evidence from reconstructions of the cranial bases of *Homo erectus* fossil skulls and fossil evidence concerning the innervation of the muscles of the thorax that permit the fine control of breathing needed for effective production of speech. The recent discovery in Java of a *Homo erectus* skull with a fairly complete basicranium has called this interpretation into question, and the proposal by Walker and Shipman concerning the innervation of the thorax of *Homo erectus* has also been criticized (Gibson, 1997). However, it is clear that, with respect to the anatomy of the hand and upper extremity, *Homo erectus* had become fully modern (Walker & Shipman, 1996; Wilson, 1998: 58).

Another hallmark of human evolution that is presumably relevant to the origin of language is the tremendous increase in brain volume, and especially the ratio of brain volume to body size, relative to the other primates, including the great apes. The oldest fossil hominid that enjoys nearly universal support by paleoanthropologists as a putative human ancestor is *Australopithecus afarensis*, dating from perhaps 4 million years ago, and having a brain no larger than that of a modern chimpanzee, perhaps 400 cc in volume. By the time of the emergence of *Homo erectus* (sometimes classified as *H. ergaster*) approximately 2 million years ago, brain volume had approximately doubled, and it had reached its current average of 1300 cc or so with the emergence of *Homo sapiens* about 200,000 years ago. What we should take from this is that increase in brain volume among the hominids was gradual, or at least step-like. It is also worth mentioning that not only was brain size increasing, but the ratios of the various parts of the brain to each other were also changing. In particular, relative to the general size of the brain, the neocortex and the cerebellum are considerably larger in humans than in apes and other primates (see Gibson & Jesse, 1999). The neocortex is generally thought to be the mediator of higher cognitive functions, including language, while the cerebellum is critical in the coordination of complex movements.

Finally, there is the question of when the cerebral asymmetry characteristic of modern humans may have arisen. This is especially important because it has been known since the mid–nineteenth century that the

human cerebral cortex is lateralized with respect to neural functions critical to the use of language. In particular, injury to two regions of the left
cerebral hemisphere, known as Broca's and Wernicke's areas after their discoverers, leads to serious disruptions of linguistic ability in most people.
It is also significant that this asymmetry for language is in some way related to human handedness, in that most people are also right-handed,
meaning that their skilled hand is also controlled by the left side of the cerebral cortex, since the motor and sensory neurons cross from one side of the
brain to the opposite side of the body. Although there is some evidence for
hand preference among chimpanzees, the degree of right-handedness
exhibited by humans is evidently unique among the primates, as are, presumably, the lateralized centers for language. It has recently been proposed,
however, that an anatomic asymmetry corresponding to Wernicke's area
can be observed in chimps post-mortem (Gannon et al., 1998), but the evidence has been questioned (see Corballis, 2002: 167, for a discussion of
the evidence). It has also been proposed (Holloway, 1983) that an anatomic
asymmetry on the left side of the brain corresponding to Broca's area is
observable in *Homo habilis*, the earliest representative of genus *Homo*,
dating to about 2.5 million years ago.

To recapitulate, the fossil evidence suggests several things concerning
the evolution of the human capacity for language. It appears to have been
incipient bipedalism and the exploitation of a more diverse ecological niche
that drove the separation of the hominids from the apes, specifically the
chimpanzees. Bipedalism has the effect of freeing the hands from constant
involvement in locomotion for other activities such as tool use and gesturing. The early hominids had brains that were not significantly larger
than those of modern chimps, and the hand began to evolve into its modern configuration at an earlier date. The characteristic human vocal apparatus probably evolved later than the hand. The brain increased in size and
organizational complexity, including its characteristic lateralization of function, fairly gradually. We suggest that this gradual evolution of the brain
argues against an abrupt appearance of fully developed language—hominids
such as *Homo erectus* that appeared long before *Homo sapiens* and had a
long and successful evolutionary history must have been using their relatively large brains for something, and we argue that some form of language,
probably gestured, must have been part of their behavioral repertoire.

2 Evidence from the Behavior
of Nonhuman Primates

There is currently no fossil evidence representing the common ancestor
of chimpanzees and humans, but if it resembled modern chimpanzees it
makes sense to assume that the behavior of chimpanzees might throw con-

siderable light on the probable behavioral capacities of the common ancestor and, thus, of the early hominids. It is well known that that chimpanzees appear quite limited in the extent to which they can learn to use spoken language (see Hayes & Nissen, 1971). There appear to be at least three possible limiting factors: anatomical, neurological, and intellectual. Anatomically speaking, it appears that the conformation of the chimpanzee vocal tract severely limits the range of sounds that can be produced (Lieberman, 1991); and from a neurological perspective, it has been maintained that nonhuman primates, including chimpanzees, lack voluntary control over their vocalizations (Myers, 1976; and see Corballis, 2002: 138). Although both of these claims have been challenged (Gibson, 1997; Steklis, 1985), chimpanzees do not appear capable of acquiring speech to a substantial degree. The question of the intellectual capabilities of chimpanzees with respect to the acquisition of speech (this is of course ultimately a neurological issue also) is much more difficult to assess, for it appears that chimpanzees are capable of comprehending speech to a much greater extent than they can produce it (see Savage-Rumbaugh, 1999). In any event, the capacity of chimpanzees, and other apes for that matter, to acquire language in a visible-gestural mode appears much greater.

With respect to vocal communication by chimpanzees in the wild, it has often been maintained that it is highly invariant and stimulus bound (see Corballis, 2002: 138). There have been recent challenges to these assertions as well. King has recently reviewed the evidence concerning this issue and comes to the following conclusion (2003: 77):

> A number of primate species [do] exhibit referential calls, as noted in a chart compiled by Hauser (1996: 520–521) in his encyclopedic work on the evolution of communication; some examples are well cited and well discussed in the primate literature, including rhesus macaque screams made by juveniles engaged in fights. These screams refer to specific aspects of the juveniles' opponents, including kinship relation and dominance level.

She goes on to note that only one of the items listed by Hauser concerns referential signaling by great apes but that the preponderance of the evidence suggests that nonhuman primates are capable of more than the "involuntary grunts and cries" mentioned by Corballis (2002: 138) as characterizing their vocal communication. King also cites research by Mitani and Gros-Louis (1998) on chimpanzee pant-hoots that "tells us that the structure of the calls as well as the rate of vocalizing may be altered according to social context" (King, 2003: 77), and she cites work by Boesch and Boesch-Achermann (2000) that identified idiosyncratic features of pant-hoots among wild chimpanzees in the Ivory Coast. Nevertheless, as we noted, the potential for linguistic behavior by the apes appears greater in the visual-gestural medium than in the vocal.

Soon after the appearance of Stokoe's initial work on ASL, it occurred to researchers that sign language might provide a better test case than speech with respect to the linguistic capacities of higher primates and, thus, those of ancestral humans. Experiments have been carried out with chimpanzees, gorillas, and the next group of Hominoidea in terms of closeness of relatedness to humans, orangutans (see Fouts & Mills, 1997; Gardner, Gardner, & Van Cantfort, 1989; Wallman, 1992). This research has been controversial with respect to what it demonstrates about the capacity of apes to acquire human language in its fullest sense, especially with respect to the acquisition of syntax. There are also important differences between apes and humans with respect to the anatomy of the hand and, therefore, the ability of apes, including chimpanzees, to form all of the handshapes of a human sign language such as ASL (see Wilson, 1998: 21–34). Nevertheless, it is clear that apes, and especially chimpanzees, can acquire a substantial vocabulary of signs, and that they can use these signs to communicate productively with human beings and, at least in the case of chimpanzees, with other apes.

It is important also to look at the capacity of apes, especially chimpanzees, to produce and comprehend motivated, that is, iconic or indexic, gestures that they have *not* been taught by human beings, in captivity and in the wild. Burling (1999: 336–340) reviews the evidence for motivated signs, generally iconic manual signs, observed among captive chimpanzees and gorillas. This includes effective gestural communication used by Viki, the chimpanzee raised by the Hayes family, who famously did not learn to speak (Hayes & Nissen, 1971); a gorilla observed using iconic gestures under naturalistic conditions at the San Francisco zoo (Tanner & Byrne, 1996); and gestures used by Kanzi and other chimpanzees studied by Savage-Rumbaugh (see Savage-Rumbaugh, 1999). Tomasello and his colleagues (1997) compiled a list of 30 gestures used by a group of captive chimpanzees at the Yerkes Primate Center. In addition to the work reviewed by Burling, there is a report of spontaneous referential pointing behavior in a captive chimpanzee (Leavens, Hopkins, & Bard, 1996), and Corballis (2003) cites other evidence of pointing by bonobos and chimps (Inoue-Nakamura & Matsuzawa, 1997; Veà & Sabater-Pi, 1998).

As Burling (1999: 339) points out, "almost nothing is known about the use of motivated signs in the wild." Although primatologists studying the behavior of chimpanzees have devoted a good deal of time to vocal behavior, it may be that until recently little attention has been given to visible gestures. Nevertheless, even cursory examination of films and photographs made by Jane Goodall, at the Gombe Stream Reserve, reveals that a wealth of communicative gestures, such as those for begging and dominance or submission, have been used by these feral chimpanzees; and many of these gestures are quite transparent to human observers (e.g., van Lawick-Goodall, 1976).

Behavioral primatologists have recently begun to give more serious consideration to the gestural behavior of both captive and wild chimpanzees. Perhaps most important in this regard is the emergence of the notion that what has been lacking is an approach to understanding the highly complex social communication of chimpanzees and gorillas—an approach more like ethnography than experimentation. Savage-Rumbaugh (1999) has made this point, but it has been best developed recently by the psychologist and philosopher Stuart Shanker and the anthropologist Barbara King (Shanker & King, 2002).

Shanker and King (2002) argue that research on the communication abilities of apes needs to shift from what they call an information-processing to a dynamic-systems model. The shift would be away from a simple sender-receiver model to increasing attention to the complexities of the interactions that take place during communicative events themselves. This is the only way to understand the intentionality of the interactions.

It is impossible to know what goes on inside an ape's head when it engages in communicative behavior with other apes or with human beings. Critics of Ape Language Research (ALR) generally raise this issue and go beyond it by asserting that apes cannot have the sort of mental representation systems that are presumably required to support the use of language. Understanding these putative systems in human beings, of course, has been a major goal of cognitive science. Shanker and King want to move us beyond this epistemological barrier by proposing that at, some level, the question is irrelevant. This may be especially true for those of us interested in how the communicative behavior of apes bears on the origins of human language. We will never know what went on inside the heads of australopithecines or early representatives of genus *Homo* either, but it is vitally important to know what sorts of behaviors these hominids might have been capable of, and ALR can help us to establish a baseline.

In proposing that we move from an information-processing to a dynamic—systems paradigm, Shanker and King are also hinting at a methodological shift in ALR from formal experimentation to ethnography as the principal means of gathering data, a position that Savage-Rumbaugh has argued forcefully (1999). Ethnography is here construed as "participant observation." We may not be able to get inside the ape's head, but at least we can enter into its social circle in a meaningful way, and that is the location from which shared meaning emerges. It is only by interacting with another human being or with an ape that we can begin to judge what our interlocutor "means" by his or her communication. As Shanker and King put it (2002: 623), when evaluating Kanzi's appropriate responses to complex requests: "This behavior just is what is called 'understanding the request.'" For many years now, anthropology has insisted that a great deal of this sort of interaction precede any judgments about the language and culture of exotic groups of humans.

How do we perceive apes, how do we judge *their* behavior, and why are these questions important? Consider this quotation from Sapir on the signed languages of the deaf that we presented in chapter 1 (1921: 21):

> Still another interesting group of transfers are the different gesture languages, developed for the use of deaf-mutes, of Trappist monks vowed to perpetual silence, or of communicating parties that are within seeing distance of each other but are out of earshot. Some of these systems are one-to-one equivalences of the normal system of speech; others, like military gesture-symbolism or the gesture language of the Plains Indians of North America (understood by tribes of mutually unintelligible forms of speech) are imperfect transfers, limiting themselves to the rendering of such grosser speech elements as are an imperative minimum under difficult circumstances.

In order to overcome prejudices like this, an early goal of sign language linguistics was to prove to a skeptical world that these languages of the deaf were full-fledged human languages, and the early descriptions of them tended to stress their structural similarities to speech, while asserting that they were not simply codes for particular spoken languages (see Taub, 2001: 3). In a linguistics dominated by the generative approach, this was taken as further proof of the existence of universal grammar, because these languages were expressed in a novel medium.

It was only possible to learn how non-Western societies actually functioned by going out and participating in them *in situ*. And only the involvement of linguists fluent in sign, including deaf signers, could lead to the fuller and richer descriptions of signed languages and their cognitive and neural underpinnings that are now emerging (Emmorey, 2002; Taub, 2001; Wilcox, 2000). If we had accepted the prejudgments of Sapir, we would not have bothered to study these languages in the first place, and if we had accepted the prejudgments of a later generation of grammarians, there would have been no need to study them in depth, because we could have assumed that they were simply products of universal grammar, hence just like spoken languages. The truth has turned out to be vastly richer and more interesting than either of these sorts of assumptions would have led us to believe.

Non-Western people and deaf people living in industrial societies are all members of species *Homo sapiens*, and we *should* be willing to license their communicative behavior as linguistic. But we should recognize, by the same token, that it is only fairly recently that the human "sciences," as developed by Westerners, have been willing to so license their behavior. Previously, their behavior, communicative and otherwise, was dismissed as inferior, and it was easy for European scholars to find justifications for this. So we should be suspicious of similar offhand dismissals of the behavior of animals that are as closely related to us as chimpanzees (see, e.g. Pinker, 1994), and here we point the interested reader to Barbara King's recent book-length account (2004) of the rich gestural behavior of captive gorillas and other apes, and the bearing of this research on gestural origin theory.

3 Monkey See, Monkey Do: The Nature of the Neurological Evidence

An overview of the behavioral as well as the neurological evidence suggests that there is a tight linkage in the brain between neurological centers that control speech and signing (see e.g., Kimura, 1993; Petitto et al., 2000). While this does not provide direct evidence for the primacy of signing in evolution, it does suggest at least parallel evolution for speech and sign. Moreover, there is recent evidence for the existence of so-called mirror neurons in the brains of nonhuman primates, specifically in the premotor cortex of monkeys, presumed by their discoverers to be an area that is homologous with Broca's area in humans (Rizzolatti & Arbib, 1998). According to Rizzolatti and Arbib, these are neurons that fire both when a monkey observes and when it performs certain specific manual activities. This suggests the existence of a neurological system in nonhuman primates that was primed to allow for the mental representation of gestural signs—the recognition that such activity can be communicative as well as instrumental.

Rizzolatti and Arbib suggest that the region of the monkey brain that contains mirror neurons may be homologous with Broca's area in humans and that there is evidence for the presence of mirror neurons in humans (which would suggest that they must be present in apes also). This would be highly significant if true. It would suggest specifically that the brain region in humans that provides the sine qua non for speech may have started out subserving instrumental manual activities that became gestural and communicative. Corballis (2002) has recently worked out in detail some of the consequences this arrangement might have for the gestural theory of language origins. Corballis is concerned especially with the lateralization of language and handedness for skilled activities to the same side of the human brain (generally the left) since there is no obvious connection between the two functions, other than, perhaps, some general gain in efficiency related to the production of rapid, sequential movements.

Corballis (2002: 166–167) points out that, although handedness to the degree characteristic of humans is quite unprecedented in the primate order (in fact in the animal kingdom), brain laterality for vocal production and comprehension is in fact fairly common among the vertebrates. He sug-

· gests that the human language capacity evolved first in the gestural mode with mirror neurons providing the neural platform, but that at this point it was bilaterally distributed in the brain. Over time, vocalization was recruited into this system until it came to predominate. Vocal communication systems tend to be lateralized, and human speech was not different in this regard. Finally, because speech was associated with manual gesture, lateralization for skilled activities was established genetically also. With respect to the evolutionary timing of the development of cerebral laterality, we pointed out earlier that claims have been made for the presence of an anatomical asymmetry corresponding to Broca's area in endocasts made from the skull of *Homo habilis* (Holloway, 1983). Moreover, there is recent evidence that an anatomic asymmetry (on the left side of the brain) is present in chimpanzees in regions homologous with Broca's area (Cantalupo & Hopkins, 2001) and Wernicke's area (Gannon et al., 1998).

We should also mention two additional neurological peculiarities of human beings. The first is an experimental illusion called the McGurk effect (McGurk & MacDonald, 1976). In this situation, a subject is shown on video a mouth articulating a particular speech sound with a different actual sound dubbed over it. Subjects will respond that they *heard* a sound different from what they actually heard—the visual experience influenced the auditory. The obvious conclusion is that the visual gesture (the mouthing) has a direct impact on the neurological decoding for audition, a quite unexpected result unless we assume that visual gesture also has some sort of precedence in our evolutionary history. Second is evidence concerning development of visual control of reaching and grasping in human infants. Visual control of reaching and grasping can be considered the second of several milestones in the development of human visual attention (Atkinson, 2000: 35–37), and it comes very early in life. The module controlling this behavior can be linked to the "mirror" neurons in the parietal-frontal cortices of nonhuman primates identified by Rizzolatti and his colleagues (1997) that were described earlier. According to Atkinson (2000: 132), "we can speculate that systems, analogous to those found in the parietal-frontal circuits of primates for gauging 'graspability' and programming reaches, first start to operate at about 7–9 months of age." We find it highly significant, with respect to the evolution of the neural underpinnings of language, that these neural circuits with a long history in the primate order are activated just before the onset of language acquisition.

Finally, it is worth discussing the acquisition of language by deaf and hearing children. There have been persistent claims that the production of manual signs by deaf and hearing children of deaf parents actually begins several months earlier than the production of speech by hearing children (see Schick, 2003: 221 for a summary), although it is difficult to separate the production of first signs from the early production of communicative gestures that is characteristic of all children. Either way, communicative gestures appear to precede the production of speech in the linguistic development of all children.

4 An Evolutionary Scenario

In summary, the evidence reviewed here suggests the following scenario. The common ancestor of chimpanzees and humans probably had a limited, but highly significant, vocal repertoire and a more substantial capacity for communication involving visible gesture, including iconic and indexic gestures. During the course of hominid evolution, the hand and upper extremity reached their modern configurations long before the upper respiratory system, including the vocal tract, did so. From this evidence, it is reasonable to conclude that the earliest language-like behavior of the hominids involved visible, especially iconic and indexic, manual signs, although vocalization was probably always an important part of the hominid communication package. There is also reason to believe that grammar, especially syntax, evolved out of iconic manual gestures.

The question of the place of syntax in the evolution of the human capacity for language has recently been reconsidered by Ray Jackendoff (2002), a leading proponent of the generative approach to linguistics. The physical anthropologist Terrence Deacon (1997) has also been critical of this focus on syntax, as has one of the authors of this book (Armstrong, 1999, refers to the problem as "syntaxophilia," but we feel that Jackendoff's term is more apt). Jackendoff uses the term "syntactocentrism" to refer to the preoccupation by generativists with syntax as the key, defining feature of human evolution, and he neatly describes the problem that this introduces for students of human evolution in terms of the classic "chicken and egg" conundrum (2003: 662):

> In the syntactocentric architecture, everything depends on
> syntax. Meaning cannot have evolved before syntax, because its
> structure is totally dependent on the syntactic structure from
> which it is derived. For the same reason, phonological structure
> cannot have evolved before syntax. Thus the complexity of
> syntax had to evolve before the complexity of the other compo-
> nents. But what would confer an adaptive advantage on a
> syntactic faculty that just generated meaningless and impercep-
> tible syntactic structures? And what would enable children to
> acquire such syntactic structures if there were no perceptible
> output to which they could attach it? We quickly see that, at
> this very crude level at least, the syntactocentric theory is
> stuck: there is no logical way to build it incrementally, such
> that the earlier stages are useful.

Jackendoff's solution to the problem is to introduce "parallel architecture"—three generative systems, phonological, semantic, and syntactic, evolving simultaneously with interface components.

At this point, while agreeing with Jackendoff about the need to move beyond syntactocentrism, we would prefer to invoke Occam's razor in terms of Stokoe's semantic phonology (see chapter 1). Stokoe proposes that the three generative systems actually emerge naturally all at once if we assume that the first linguistic units were iconic manual gestures, such as the "grasp" gesture in which one open hand sweeps in front of the chest and seizes the upright index finger of the other hand (1991: 112):

> An *s-p* [semantic-phonological] *noun-verb* unit represents a
> word of sign language, it is both an agent-verb construct and in
> the lexicon a formal noun or verb or other part of speech of the
> language, and it can combine in the normal way with others
> like it to make a grammatical noun-verb structure. This struc
> ture in turn has meaning (actually it always had).

Stokoe here discusses the recursive nature of the elementary syntactic-semantic unit that makes up such a manual gesture, but he indicates also that these gestures contain the elements of the phonological system as well (hence semantic phonology) in terms of the elementary handshapes and movements that become the components of a true signed language, once the hominids who used them recognized that they had a componential structure and thus could be decomposed and recombined. There is thus no need, at least at the earliest stages of language evolution, to invoke the three separately evolving systems Jackendoff proposes—when we view iconic manual gestures in this way, the whole seamless system can be seen to appear at once.

It seems to us that what is needed beyond this point in the evolutionary history of the hominids is progressive elaboration of the system, which is accomplished essentially by grammaticalization—the process by which grammatical structures develop and evolve. This, in turn, can be seen to involve a variety of metaphorical processes. In the remainder of this book, we intend to work out the implications of this claim in terms of the evolution of signed languages. Our most significant claim is that the processes at work in the elaboration of signed languages are analogous to what occurred and continues to occur in the evolution of speech. We will show that the advantage of taking signed languages as a starting point is that these processes of evolution are much more transparent and easily construed in sign than in speech. We end this chapter with an example of the metaphorical processes at work in the grammaticalization of a sign language from a recent book by Phyllis Perrin Wilcox (2000).

Wilcox is especially interested in how such metaphorical mappings result in grammaticalization, the process by which grammatical forms emerge out of lexical items. In pursuit of this goal, Wilcox conducts a detailed historical analysis of the ASL sign GIVE, tracing it to its roots in French Sign Language (LSF). It is possible to make this connection because it is known, as we will show in chapter 7, that ASL was heavily influenced in its development for educational purposes by LSF.

Wilcox shows how what may have begun as an iconic sign for a French coin ultimately, through metaphorical extension, becomes an ASL discourse marker, GIVE-*concede*, meaning, roughly, "I give up, you win the argument." According to Wilcox's analysis,

> tracking the ASL sign GIVE and its variants reveals a coherent
> path of lexicalization: (1) a noun representing an old French
> coin; (2) related LSF verbs, adjectives, and nouns having to do
> with money exchange; (3) ASL giving constructions of classifiers
> and frozen conventionalization; (4) ASL signs having to do with
> permanent possession, money, and value; (5) metaphorical
> extensions of literal giving verbs; (6) a regional offshoot adjective
> variant with its underlying sense of money (CROOK); and finally
> (7) the wholly metaphorical $GIVE_2$-*concede*. This path of
> lexicalization provides evidence of potential grammaticalization
> of GIVE in ASL. (2000: 168–169)

With regard to the metaphorical basis of grammaticalization, similar processes may be at work in both signed and spoken languages. For example, in ASL and some other signed languages, the future is indicated as the space in front of the signer and the past by the space behind. Armstrong, Stokoe, and Wilcox (1995: 122) point out that this "can be translated into the 'grammar' of locomotion. The space in front of the signer is where he or she will be in the future and the space behind is where he or she was in the past." Exactly the same metaphorical process was at work in the development of the English construction "am gonna" to indicate future tense, as in "I'm gonna wake up at ten tomorrow morning." As the language evolved, a construction indicating movement through space—"I'm going to St. Ives"—came to indicate "movement" through time.

We think that it is possible to show processes like these at work pervasively in the development of signed languages, and in the next chapter we expand on this theme. In particular, we explore the iconic relationships underlying grammatical constructions in these languages that have been called "classifier constructions" or "classifier predicates." In addition, we consider evidence concerning the neural mechanisms in the brain that make it possible for human beings to employ these highly complex iconic processes as they develop languages.

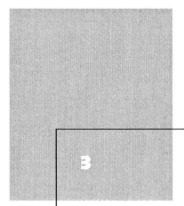

THREE

Gesture, Sign, and Speech

1 The Domain of Gesture

As Kendon (2000) notes, how we view the relation between language and gesture depends on how the two are defined. The challenge is to not simply define language and gesture as the same thing, or to define them as essentially different. The approach we prefer is one that recognizes what unites language, both spoken and signed, with gesture, and that also permits us to acknowledge and understand their fundamental differences.

Naturally, any definition that attempts to classify together such disparate phenomena as gestures, spoken words, and signed words must be formulated at a relatively high level of abstraction. We will use the term 'gesture' in two senses. In the first sense, we start with the definition of gesture adopted in our earlier work (e.g. Armstrong et al., 1995: 43), which follows Studdert-Kennedy's statement that "a gesture is a functional unit, an equivalence class of coordinated movements that achieve some end" (1987: 77). This definition is not intended to distinguish gestures from signs or words. Rather, it encompasses the articulatory movements that constitute spoken and signed words, as well as other functional bodily actions, whether or not they are intentionally produced or communicative. A key aspect of the definition is that it is neutral with regard to the type of function that is performed. This definition permits us to classify together for purposes of analysis actions that serve quite different functional goals. For example, this approach reveals connections between actions serving a communicative function and those serving an instrumental but noncommunicative function. Likewise, because this approach also does not require that the goal be *intentionally* achieved, it permits the study of developmental links between nonintentional and intentional functional actions. Finally, the definition does not include or exclude data on the basis of articulatory apparatus: manual, facial, postural, and other bodily actions are all included. This is essentially the position taken by phoneticians such as Björn Lindblom (1990: 220):

> Human communication . . . includes forms of verbal communication such as speech, written language and sign language. It comprises nonverbal modes that do not invoke language proper, but that nevertheless constitute extremely important aspects of how we communicate. As we interact, we make various gestures—some vocal and audible, others nonvocal like patterns of eye contact and movements of the face and the body. Whether intentional or not, these behaviors carry a great deal of communicative significance.

There are several benefits to adopting this functional definition of gesture. As Armstrong and colleagues (1995) point out, a broadly conceived, functional conception allows us to categorize together the articulatory movements of speech (Browman & Goldstein, 1989; Neisser, 1967) with cospeech gestures and the movements making up the signs of signed languages as part of a dynamic system of bodily action (Kelso, Saltzman, & Tuller, 1986; King, 2004).

In the second sense that we use the term 'gesture,' words, signs, and even meaningful, everyday gestures are regarded as manifestations of gesture in the first, articulatory sense. Words are regarded as coordinated patterns of articulatory gestures: "words are not simply strings of individual gestures, produced one after the other; rather, each is a particular pattern of gestures, orchestrated appropriately in time and space" (Kelso, Saltzman, & Tuller, 1986: 31). Signs are also regarded as coordinated patterns of articulatory gestures produced appropriately in time and space. And the body actions studied by gesture researchers such as Calbris, Kendon, McNeill, and others are treated the same way. The "Hand Purse" described by Kendon (1995) is a coordinated pattern of articulatory gestures involving the fingers, wrist, forearm, and upper arm, produced appropriately in time and space. Like spoken and signed words, such gestures are also regarded as action complexes composed of coordinated patterns of movements that achieve some end. All three—words, signs, and meaningful gestures—are made up of articulatory gestures.

The fact that words, signs, and gestures are each treated as manifestations of gesture does not prevent us from noting significant differences among them. Here, too, we prefer to take an approach that does not simply attempt to define clear-cut categories of word, sign, and gesture. Instead, we propose certain dimensions along which these phenomena vary, such as articulatory and perceptual systems, medium of transmission, conventionalization, schematicity, symbolic complexity, and autonomy-dependence.

For example, spoken and signed words are produced by different articulatory systems, are transmitted in different channels (acoustic vs. optic), and are received by different perceptual systems. While words and signs are recognized as conventionally belonging to particular linguistic systems, gestures are not. This is especially important in the case of signs, since they share articulatory and perceptual systems with gestures.

By not including intentionality or communicativeness as part of the definition of gesture, this approach permits the study of how unintentional, noncommunicative gestures may come to acquire communicative significance. Such development occurs on an evolutionary scale, such as the development of "intention movements" in animals (Krebs & Davies, 1993), as well as ontogenetically, both among nonhuman primates (Plooij, 1984) and humans (Singleton et al., 1993). Researchers such as King (2004) report that such an approach to gesture permits the exploration of how gestural communication emerges in the nonvocal social communication of African great apes.

Thus, the definition of gesture adopted here has a methodological motivation. In the early stages of conceptualizing the role that visible gesture might play in the evolution of language, it is important that we do not make arbitrary distinctions. The functional definition adopted here allows us to categorize together disparate phenomena and understand them as manifestations of a common underlying system—it facilitates the search for an overarching theory of communication by means of bodily action. This overarching theory recognizes that language, too, has its precursors, in several senses. First, unless we accept a discontinuity hypothesis and assume that language began with an unexplainable "big bang," we must search for the evolutionary precursors to language. An increasing number of researchers point to gesture as this precursor (Arbib & Rizzolatti, 1996; Armstrong, 1999; Armstrong, Stokoe, & Wilcox, 1994, 1995; Armstrong & Wilcox, 2002; Corballis, 2002; Hewes, 1992; Kimura, 1993; King, 1999, 2004; Rizzolatti & Arbib, 1998; Stokoe, 2001).

Second, evidence points to visible gesture as an ontogenetic precursor to language (Blake, 2000; Blake & Dolgoy, 1993; Capirci et al., 2002). Although not specifically addressing gesture, Haiman (1998a) suggests that these two courses of development are manifestations of ritualization, whereby instrumental actions are transformed into symbolic actions, and proposes that ritualization can account for the emergence of language from nonlanguage (128):

> The . . . evolution of language from originally instrumental
> action to symbolic is plausible: elsewhere in the animal
> kingdom, semanticization or emancipation occurred wherever
> originally instrumental acts were modified and stylized to
> produce signals.

We will present our own theory about the role of ritualization in the emergence of language in chapter 4.

There is a third sense in which language has precursors. Linguists have identified a process called grammaticization by which grammatical morphemes gradually develop from lexical morphemes or a combination of lexical morphemes with lexical or grammatical morphemes (Bybee, Perkins, & Pagliuca, 1994: 4). We will examine the gestural precursors of language in this third sense in chapter 6, where we propose that the cognitive and social processes that drive grammaticization also account for the development of language from gesture.

2 Speech as Gesture

If visible gesture played a critical role in the origin of human language, it is reasonable to ask why human language is now predominantly spoken, with signed languages being used only among certain special populations. The question is typically seen as dealing with the transition from gesture to spoken language; however, this conception of the problem is flawed in at least two ways.

First, as our discussion of the domain of gesture makes clear, we regard all language as ultimately gestural: certain parts of the body move in a way that produces a signal. Signed languages are articulated by moving hands, face, and body to produce an optical signal that is received by the visual perceptual system. Spoken languages are articulated by moving parts of the vocal tract to produce an acoustic signal that is received by the auditory perceptual system. As the cognitive psychologist Ulric Neisser noted (1967: 156):

> To speak is to make finely controlled movements in certain parts
> of your body, with the result that information about these
> movements is broadcast to the environment. For this reason the
> movements of speech are sometimes called *articulatory gestures*.
> A person who perceives speech, then, is picking up information
> about a certain class of real, physical, tangible . . . events.

Whether the activity is speaking or signing, and whether the signal produced is audible or visible, the events in question are fundamentally gestural.

Second, this view of language origins does not require a transition from a period in which human ancestors used only visible gestures to one in which modern humans use only acoustic gestures. At no time in our entire evolutionary history did communication take place in a single modality. Modern primates are active vocalizers but also active gesturers. The evidence is also quite clear that humans gesture while they vocalize. The evolutionary link between gesture and language is so strong that even congenitally blind people who have never seen visible gesture nevertheless produce gestures when speaking with each other (Iverson, 1998). On the basis of the body of research on gesture and language, McNeill has concluded that "gestures and speech should be viewed within a unified conceptual framework as aspects of a single underlying process" (1992: 23).

The picture that emerges is thus one in which both visible and acoustic gestures played an early role in hominid communication and continue to be primary means by which humans communicate today. What has changed is the relative informational load carried by visible versus audible gestures. Visible gesture is clearly implicated as playing a critical role in the early evolutionary history of language. It is also evident that at some point, natural selection favored acoustic gestures as the primary means by which information is broadcast to the environment for purposes of linguistic communication, at least among hearing communities.

In spite of this shift in the balance of informational load, visible gesture remains a significant part of the overall human communication system, suggesting a single, unified system. Gesture also remains in other facets of signed and spoken language. Dwight Bolinger, for example, posited a "gestural complex that includes intonation" (1986: 197), suggesting that this gestural complex reflects an ancient mixed system of gesture and speech. Bolinger even went so far as to suggest that this mixed system survives today, though gesture and intonation have evolved along somewhat separate paths (198). In support of this suggestion he cites Kendon, who notes that speech and gesture are so intricately coordinated that "it is as if the speech production process is manifested in two forms of activity simultaneously: in the vocal organs and also in bodily movement" (1980: 211). However, since vocal organ activity is also bodily movement, only *one* form of gestural activity needs to be posited. Finally, gesture remains even in signed languages. A growing body of research is now examining the gesture-language interface in signed languages (Emmorey & Riley, 1995; Liddell, 1998, 2003; Liddell & Metzger, 1998; Morford & Kegl, 2000).

We will explore this interface, including whether or not there really is such an interface or whether we are simply talking about a continuum of structures that range from the iconic and analogous to the arbitrary and digital, in more detail in the next section, but first we return to the question we posed in the opening paragraph of this section: If visible gesture played a critical role in the origin of human language, a reasonable question to ask is why human language is now predominantly spoken.

Anyone who speculates that human language was once carried primarily in the visible-gestural channel must account for why speech would eventually come to predominate. A number of writers have addressed this issue, including one of us (Armstrong, 1999), and Corballis (2002: 186–198) has recently summarized much of the speculation. A list of the usual suspects follows: speech may be more energy efficient than signing; speech frees the hands for tool use and for demonstration of other manual techniques to novices; speech is effective in the dark and past opaque obstacles; hearing does not require directed attention as does vision. We will devote more attention to this issue in chapter 4, but here we note that there is some highly interesting evidence that the transition to fully articulate speech may have been a fairly recent occurrence in human evolutionary history. This evidence is provided by what has been named the FOXP2 gene.

FOXP2 is one of a number of genes that have recently been identified as having an important role in the differentiation of chimps and humans (see Pennisi, 2006). A genetic disorder at first thought to affect only grammatical processing (Gopnick, 1990) and later shown to affect other aspects of language, including movements of the facial and oral musculature (Fisher et al., 1998), has been linked to this regulatory gene (Lai et al., 2001). It has recently been shown (Enard et al., 2002) that this gene has undergone relatively extensive evolution in the hominid lineage since its split with chimpanzees, and that, in particular, a mutation that favored articulate speech was probably fixed in the human population as recently as only one hundred to two hundred thousand years ago, or perhaps coincident with the appearance of modern *Homo sapiens*. A reasonable interpretation of the function of this gene in its modern human form is that it was the final piece in a genetic mosaic that made articulate speech efficient and useable as the primary channel for human language (see Balter, 2002). Because, as we noted previously, the brain had already achieved its modern size and form by the time this gene emerged in its modern form, it is also reasonable to propose that well—developed sign languages had already been in use well before this, and that the human FOXP2 mutation simply enabled a shift to speech for adaptive reasons that were outlined in the previous paragraph.

3 Speech and Sign

As we pointed out, it may be fruitful to think of signed languages as gestural systems with aspects of their grammars having analog features. In particular, it may be interesting to think about what have been called classifier constructions in this regard (we will return to these signed linguistic devices in chapter 5), and we will be drawing here on a recent comprehensive review of the literature on classifier constructions and their neurological representation by Emmorey (2002).

According to Emmorey,

> classifier constructions are the primary linguistic structures used to express both concrete and abstract concepts of motion and location. ASL signers also exploit signing space to schematically represent spatial relations, time, and aspects of conceptual structure. When signers describe spatial relations, there is a structural analogy between the form of a classifier construction and aspects of the described scene. (2002: 115)

In other words, the nature of the structural relationship between the form of the signed utterance and the described scene is generally iconic (either directly or by metaphoric extension). The idea that ASL grammar is at least partly analog is not new (e.g., DeMatteo, 1977), and it has been hotly contested. What is now possible, and what Emmorey does, is give us a comprehensive account of the interplay of analog and digital processes in ASL and the consequences of this complexity for both language acquisition by children and the consequent representation of these processes in the brain.

In fact, what Emmorey makes clear is that far from marking ASL as simpler or more primitive than speech, an old prejudice, analog processes such as classifier constructions may be extremely complex and difficult to acquire:

> In sum, children do not acquire the ASL classifier system easily or without error, despite the clear iconicity of the system. At the youngest ages (2;0 to 3;0), children are able to produce handling classifier handshapes and use whole entity classifier handshapes to designate a moving figure object. However, the ability to integrate the use of the hands to express figure and ground relationships is not fully developed until late in childhood. Furthermore, learning the language-specific constraints on the combination of classifier handshapes and movement components occurs throughout childhood. Thus, unlike speaking children, who may produce early gestures that resemble classifier constructions, signing children are acquiring a linguistic system of contrasts in which the phonological, morphological, and semantic-pragmatic properties of classifier forms must be learned. (2002: 198)

But there is more going on here than linguistic (especially phono-logical) encoding, and it may be the interplay of what look like fully phonemicized aspects of signing (e.g., handshapes) and what look like gestural elements (e.g., pointing and directed movements) that makes signed languages so hard to learn. According to Liddell,

> signers know where things are and direct signs toward them
> through the ability to point. The handshapes, orientation of the
> hand(s), the type of movement (straight, arc) are linguistically
> defined. The directionality of the signs is not linguistically
> defined. It is variable, depending completely on the actual or
> conceptualized location of the entity the sign is directed toward.
> . . . There are more than fifteen distinct proposals attempting
> to provide grammatical explanations for verb directionality.
> Only one, Liddell and Johnson (1989), attempts to provide a
> phonological system capable of encoding spatial loci. Even this
> complex system is inadequate to the task. (2002: 75)

According to Emmorey, classifier constructions can be defined as "com-plex predicates that express *motion, position, stative-descriptive,* and *han-dling* information" (73–74). Figure 3.1 illustrates how classifiers work in ASL. In this example, a picture hanging on a wall is represented by the signer's diagramming a square in front of his face, and the event of the picture shifting its position is shown by a different set of handshapes, as is the act of returning the picture to its original position.

Emmorey (2002) presents comprehensive information on the neurologi-cal representation of classifier constructions in ASL. There is abundant evi-dence, as we have seen, that both speech and sign are critically dependent on structures generally located in the cortex of the left cerebral hemisphere, structures traditionally known as Broca's and Wernicke's areas. It is critical to an understanding of the nature of language and its genetic underpinnings to know why these languages in radically different perceptual modes share the same neurological platform. Is this due to genetic determination for universal grammar or could it be due to factors related to underlying simi-larities in processing and production—particularly the reliance by both sys-tems on the decoding and production of rapid sequential movements? And perhaps more interesting, are there differences in neurological representa-tion between speech and sign at the cerebral hemispheric level?

Emmorey reviews the available evidence (much expanded due to the rapid proliferation of brain imaging technology) bearing on these questions and concludes that

> both neural plasticity and rigidity are observed for the neural
> organization within the left hemisphere for Deaf signers. Neural

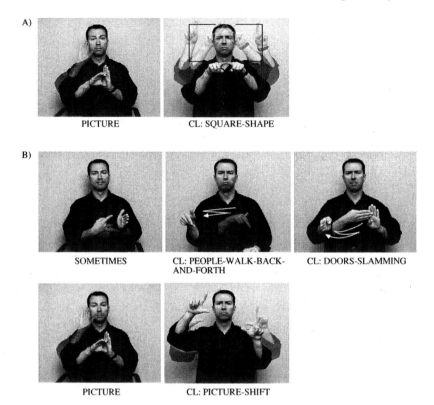

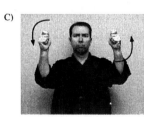

Figure 3.1. Classifier use in ASL. The discourse could be interpreted as (A) "The picture is square," (B) "Sometimes when people walk by and doors slam, the picture can shift position," and (C) "You simply readjust the picture." From Karen Emmorey, *Language, Cognition, and the Brain: Insights from Sign Language* (Mahwah, NJ: Erlbaum), page 75. © 2002 by Lawrence Erlbaum Associates. Reproduced here with the permission of the publisher.

plasticity is observed for auditory related cortex, which has
received little or no auditory input, but nonetheless is engaged
in processing the visual input of sign language. More striking,
perhaps, is that the same neural structures (e.g., Broca's area,
Wernicke's area) are engaged for the production and comprehension of both signed and spoken language. This neural
invariance across language modalities points to a biological or
developmental bias for these neural structures to mediate
language at a more abstract level, divorced from the sensory
and motoric systems that perceive and transmit language.
(2002: 313)

In support of these conclusions, Emmorey cites evidence for the dissociation of sign language and symbolic gesture. It is the case, however, as
Emmorey points out, that "it is unlikely that motor planning for signing is
completely autonomous and independent of the motor planning systems
involved in nonlinguistic movements" (2002: 283).

As we mentioned, given the uniqueness of the classifier constructions,
their neural representation should prove instructive. If they are only partially phonemicized (i.e., dependent on sequentially arranged and discrete
abstract units) and heavily dependent on perception and manipulation of
three-dimensional space, we might expect that there would be right cerebral hemispheric involvement in their processing. Emmorey indicates that
this may be the case (2002: 313):

There is currently some controversy regarding the role of the
right hemisphere in sign language processing. . . . At least one
functional brain imaging study revealed a large amount of right
hemisphere activity during sign language comprehension.
Whether this degree of right-hemisphere activation is similar to
that observed during spoken language processing remains to be
seen. For both spoken and signed language comprehension, the
right hemisphere appears to be involved in processing some
discourse-level functions. . . . Nonetheless, for sign language,
the right hemisphere may play a unique role in the production
and comprehension of the topographic functions of signing
space, particularly as conveyed by classifier constructions.

The prospect that brain imaging studies of sign language users may
help to resolve some of these questions suggests an exciting near—term
future for study in this area.

Equally interesting is Emmorey's treatment of the structure of working memory for ASL. Here she summarizes evidence, much of it from her
own recent research, concerning the structural similarities in working

memory for signed and spoken languages, but also an intriguing difference that may be modality specific. Working memory for sign and speech appears to make use of phonological coding, but

> sign-based and speech-based working memory each take advantage of the distinctive capacities of their respective sensory modalities. Audition appears to be particularly well suited for retaining information about sequences of stimuli over time whereas vision excels at processing stimuli distinguished by spatial location. Similarly, speech based working memory appears to excel at using time to code serial order, whereas sign-based working memory is able to use space to code serial order. In addition, the distinct articulatory properties of sign and speech lead to differences in memory span, apparently due to a universal limit on the articulatory loop. (2002: 240)

With regard to this discussion of working memory, some differences between speech and sign are based on modality, but a basic structural similarity in a "peripheral" language processor suggests that sign at least co-evolved with speech if it did not precede it in human evolution. How else can we explain the use of the same architecture for both? An appeal to an abstract linguistic code as the basis seems to be undercut by the modality—based differences, and there appear to be too many details in common that are open to functional explanations for there to be simple genetic causation for "language" per se. In this regard, it is worth mentioning again, as further evidence for a signing stage in the evolution of the capacity for language, the recent evidence for late onset of speech in human evolutionary history that we discussed earlier (e.g., Balter, 2002): the so-called speech gene, FOXP2, representing a genetically based difference in control of vocal articulation between chimps and humans that may have arisen as recently as 100,000 to 200,000 years ago (with the emergence of *Homo sapiens).* Under this scenario, the neural architecture of language, involving structures such as Broca's area, originally evolved in response to the use of visible gesture, that were later coopted by speech when gene mutations made that medium available for efficient communication.

Focusing on the differences or suggesting that signing is older in the human lineage in no way implies that signed languages are simpler than or inferior to spoken languages. The complexity of spatial reference and classifier systems suggests quite the opposite. Classifier systems are rich and complex and may, in fact, make signed languages harder to master than speech. If this is true, then we can add at least two possible explanations for the current predominance of speech in human communication to those that we listed earlier—speech is inherently simpler, or human beings, as a result of using speech for some considerable period of time, have evolved special neurological mechanisms that enable it to be acquired more easily than signing.

It is impossible to say at present how much of the similarity in neurological representation between sign and speech is due to the architecture of the human nervous system's variations on the basic hominoid pattern, how much is due to human beings rediscovering basic principles that provide for the most efficiency and effectiveness within the particular modality, how much is due to coevolution of the nervous and linguistic systems, and how much is due to language-specific genetic determination.

If we assume that sign language accompanied speech in evolutionary history (or even preceded it) we do not have to see Broca's area as being uniquely modular for language—it could have been built on a practical action/communication platform à la Rizzolatti and Arbib (1998) in terms of mirror neurons. According to this scenario, the emergence of classifiers might represent the emergence of linguistic conceptualization, as humans saw that they could take apart holistic gestures and manipulate and recombine their components in terms of handshapes and movements. In Stokoe's (1991) semantic-phonological terms, these could be seen as nouns and verbs, the elements of simple sentences.

From this point of view, it is easy to move to a conception of the origin of recursion in human language. Semantic phonology suggests that language structures are built of components that are structurally identical to themselves: sign language sentences are composed of signs, but signs are composed of semantic-phonological "sentences" or *noun-verb* constructions. This quality of visible gesture can be thought of as recursive, because "recursive structures are built of components that are structurally identical to themselves" (Gelernter, 1998: 58). When we think of recursion in generative grammatical terms, we usually think of embedded phrases, but the notion applies equally to sign language signs embedded within longer strings that function as sentences. We propose that what is needed to "bootstrap" such constructions up into real language is a brain with substantial processing and storage capacity (i.e., a brain that is large relative to body size) and a historical development process that fits these larger constructions to the social and technological needs of human populations.

4 Visible Verbs Become Vocal

Stokoe (2001: 176–193) suggests that classifiers may be seen as forming bridges in some respects between an ancient signing past and a spoken present, and that aspects of their use in spoken languages may provide direct evidence for at least the cooccurrence of sign and speech in evolutionary history, if not for the precedence of signing. The iconic manual classifier constructions (sometimes referred to as classifier predicates) described earlier have direct analogs in the morphological processes of many spoken languages, including some Native American languages, such as Navajo, that have been termed "classifier languages" (Allan, 1977). According to Allan,

> classifiers are defined on two criteria: (a) they occur as mor-
> phemes in surface structures under specifiable conditions; (b)
> they have meaning, in the sense that a classifier denotes some
> salient perceived or imputed characteristic of the entity to
> which an associated noun refers (or may refer). (285)

We have already seen that the representation of certain characteristics of nouns in ASL may be accomplished iconically by handshapes, as illustrated in figure 3.1. A wide range of such representations is possible for objects with cylindrical or long narrow shapes or square shapes, and so on.

In a spoken language like Navajo, the classification is accomplished with a noniconic spoken morpheme. According to Kluckhohn and Leighton, Navajo verbs have different stems depending on the type of object with respect to which the verb is expressing action or state: "the long-object class (a pencil, a stick, a pipe); the slender-flexible-object class (snakes, thongs, certain pluralities including certain types of food and property); the container-*and*-contents class; the granular-mass class (sugar, salt, etc.); the things-bundled-up class (hay, bundles of clothing, etc.—if they are loose and not compact) . . . and others" (1951: 191). Of course, many of these classes of objects have parallels in the classifier systems of signed languages such as ASL.

Stokoe suggests that the existence of classifier systems in spoken languages is evidence for direct transfer of signed grammatical forms into speech. Referring to two Native languages of the American Northwest, he writes:

> Because many sign language verbs represent what they mean
> naturally and directly, and because the structure of certain
> Klamath and Modoc verbs is exactly the structure of these
> natural gestures and sign language verbs, it follows that the
> vocal representations began as a literal translation of the visible
> action. The alternative—that the gestures were intentionally
> made to copy the structure of the spoken verbs—is absurd.
> (2001: 180)

In support of this conclusion, Stokoe (2001: 184–185) points out that classifiers that occur in spoken languages can refer to a variety of qualities of objects and their actions, including: material, shape, consistency, size, location, arrangement, and quanta; but they never refer to color. He points out that although color is visible, it cannot be represented through direct iconicity in a signed language, thus was not available for translation into speech. In a signed language like ASL, color can be indicated indexically by pointing, for example, to the eyebrow to signify black, or it may reproduce the sign for an object with a distinctive color, such as orange; but there is no way to represent color on the hands or body through direct iconicity.

It is worth noting here that there is reason to believe that, as the societies that particular languages support become more complex and the communities of their speakers expand, the morphological processes that support functions like classification tend to be reduced and the basic lexicon tends to expand. We have referred to this before (Armstrong, 1999: 161–162), but it bears repeating, as most linguists have shied away from relating changes in languages to changes in technology and social complexity. Armstrong and Katz (1981) provide support for the following observations by Swadesh. Swadesh (1971) identifies three stages in the growth of languages: (1) local, (2) classic, (3) world; and these correspond to stages in the development of social complexity. Again, these should not be taken as "evolutionary" stages in the sense that one form is superior to another—they appear to be simple correlations between language structures and social structures.

With respect to the development of modern world languages, Swadesh writes:

1. Internal inflections formed by consonantal vowel alternations have been lost or reduced in number. New instances of internal inflections are few and limited in scope. The old ones are generally confined to traditional elements of the language; rarely are they applied to new loan words.
2. There are more instances in which inflective categories formed by affixation are reduced in number than cases in which new categories of this type have been added. Relational particles and auxiliary words sometimes fill the function of old inflective endings. (1971: 76)

With respect to the development from local to classic languages, he adds:

The material we have surveyed . . . suggests that languages in the local stage had limited sets of phonemes available for lexical contrast, but complex patterns of alternates used in extensive paradigms of internal inflection; that the lexicon was small and the inflection complex; and that different languages were relatively similar with regard to all these features. The development since that time has been toward a greatly increased vocabulary with a more or less drastic reduction in inflection. (Swadesh, 1971: 112)

According to Swadesh, then, in the terms of traditional structural linguistics, languages tend to become more analytic as their social circumstances become more complex—that is, languages come to rely more on grammatical words and syntactic features like word order for establishing grammatical relationships and less on morphological processes like inflections for class, person, and so on. Most linguists who have studied signed languages would classify them as highly synthetic (polysynthetic), reliant on complex morphology, and thus like Swadesh's local or classic languages.

Hymes offers a functional explanation for these trends:

Differential complexity in surface word-structure may well be adaptive, complexity being a function of boundary maintenance in the case of small communities and groups, and simplicity a function of a language's use as a lingua franca. (1971: vii)

In other words, as we suggested earlier with respect to classifiers in signed languages, extreme morphological complexity may make a language harder to learn, and thus more useful as a means for identifying in-group members, than it would be if the grammar were more analytic. The main point is that these grammatical processes are anchored in the real, visible world, and that they continue to be influenced by the forms of the human societies they serve.

Having accounted for the possibility that complex grammatical structures could evolve out of the stuff of iconic visible gesture, we move to the heart of our evolutionary argument. Ritualization is a well-known process in the study of behavioral evolution, and we employ its principles in the next chapter to show how the processes of structural change that we have discussed so far lead to the emergence of true language.

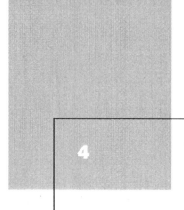

FOUR

4

Gesture, Sign, and Grammar

The Ritualization of Language

1 Gesture and the Origin of Grammar

As we noted in chapter 1, there has long been a sense that the signs of the signed languages of the deaf were somehow more "natural" than the words of spoken languages, no doubt because of their inherent iconicity. Baynton notes that sign language practitioners in the nineteenth century also saw its syntax in this way (2002: 19):

> Sign language syntax was also thought to be more natural than that of spoken languages. The Reverend Collins Stone, a teacher at the Hartford school [the American School for the Deaf], explained that sign language followed the natural order of thought rather than the "inverted and arbitrary forms of written language." Rather than the "the subject coming first, and the action, quality and object following," as in artificial languages, when the deaf person sought to express something, "the object first attracts his attention, then its qualities, and afterward the other circumstances connected with it."

This describes a form of grammatical organization that linguists have come to call topic-comment. Several decades of study have convinced linguists that the grammars of the signed languages of the deaf are fully as complex as those of spoken languages, but the idea of an analogous relationship between signed linguistic structures and what they refer to has lingered. We will give further consideration to this idea as we explore how these languages might have arisen and developed.

2 Ritual and Continuity

We take what has been called a "continuity" approach to the evolution of the capacity for language (King, 1994, 1999). This entails a theoretical appeal to evolutionary processes that transcend differences among species, in this case, species of primates. In this chapter, we take up a challenge posed by Bickerton (1995: 35): if we are to account for the evolution of language, we must have a clear understanding of what language is in all its detail, complexity, and knotty peculiarities. In addition, from our perspective, there is also a need to invoke evolutionary processes that are known to operate on animal behavior in general. Here we propose to invoke just such a process, ritualization, that is well known in ethology from pioneers in the field, including Konrad Lorenz, and we propose to apply it to what Bickerton saw as the thorniest problem of all—the evolutionary emergence of syntax.

2.1 What Is Language?

There have been many linguistic theories. Two we will discuss in depth in this chapter are the Cartesian approach (Bickerton, 1990; Chomsky, 1966; Pinker, 1994) and the cognitive approach (Lakoff, 1987; Langacker, 1987, 1988, 1991b). We focus on these two because they provide strikingly different views of what language is and how it is related to other perceptual and cognitive abilities. A third approach to language, generally called the functional approach (Bybee, Perkins, & Pagliuca, 1994; Givón, 1989, 1995; Haiman, 1985, 1994, 1998b), is also relevant to discussion of language evolution. We will explore in some detail Haiman's proposals (1994, 1998b) concerning the role of ritualization in the evolution of language.

The Cartesian approach is probably the one that is most familiar to nonlinguists, and it is the approach that many primatologists and anthropologists tend to adopt at least tacitly, if not explicitly, when they delve into the evolutionary issues involved in the study of language. Many attempts to find precursors or analogs to language abilities in modern nonhuman primates or to speculate about possible language precursors in hominid abilities and social life begin with a search for the language abilities posited by Cartesian linguists. However, the Cartesian approach, the best known modern version of which is generally called "Chomskyan" or "generative," makes inherently discontinuous assumptions at the outset. If, for example, the syntactic features of human language are unique in the animal kingdom and are tightly interwoven, how could they have arisen by stages from some previous set of conditions? Stated in those terms, the problem being posed is not different from the problem of explaining the evolution of another uniquely human trait—orthograde bipedal locomotion. The upright, striding, two-legged gait of modern humans has no analog in the animal kingdom, yet most biologically oriented scholars are willing to assume that it evolved through some set of intermediate stages, even if it has no obvious precursors among living relatives of modern humans.

Beyond the dissociation between animal communication and human language, Cartesian linguists also insist on a dissociation between general cognitive abilities and the unique, autonomous, modular language faculty. This dissociation can be traced back to Descartes's position on the relation between two modes of conceptualization: understanding, or reasoning, and imagination:

> I believe that this power of imagining that is in me, insofar as it
> differs from the power of understanding, is not a necessary
> element of my essence, that is, of the essence of my mind; for
> although I might lack this power, nonetheless I would undoubt-
> edly remain the same person I am now. Thus, it seems that the
> power of imagining depends upon something different from
> me. (Descartes, 1980 [1641]: 90)

In the Cartesian approach, language is built upon reason—the mind—not imagination (which has its basis in the body). This position on language has tremendous ramifications for how the language faculty is situated with respect to general cognitive abilities. Thus Chomsky, in his book *Cartesian Linguistics*: "In short, man has a species-specific capacity, a unique type of intellectual organization which cannot be attributed to peripheral organs or related to general intelligence and which manifests itself in what we may refer to as the 'creative aspect' of ordinary language—its property of being both unbounded in scope and stimulus-free" (1966: 4–5).

This claim, in turn, can be linked to the Cartesian position that our mental processes, our cognitive abilities, are not grounded in our bodily based perceptual or manipulative abilities:

> Although perhaps . . . I have a body that is very closely joined
> to me, nevertheless, because on the one hand I have a clear and
> distinct idea of myself—insofar as I am a thing that thinks and
> not an extended thing—and because on the other hand I have a
> distinct idea of a body—insofar as it is merely an extended

thing, and not a thing that thinks—it is therefore certain that I
am truly distinct from my body, and that I can exist without it.
(Descartes, 1980 [1641]: 93)

As we pointed out in the previous chapter, quoting Jackendoff, Cartesian linguistics considers the essence of language to be grammar, and grammar to be a self-contained system describable without reference to other
cognitive abilities—a separate mental module or faculty. The Cartesian approach treats grammar as an autonomous system distinct from both lexicon
and semantics. Under this approach, the best model for understanding this
self-contained linguistic system is that of a set of formal algorithms for gen-
erating well-formed sentences. Redundancy is avoided in describing such a
system because redundancy implies a loss of generalization, a lack of parsi-
mony; economy is a prime goal in Cartesian versions of linguistic theory.

Cognitive linguistics makes quite different assumptions about the nature of language that are much more compatible with Darwinian approaches
to language evolution. In contrast to Cartesian linguists, cognitive linguists insist that language relies on general cognitive abilities. The goal
of cognitive linguistics is to determine what these abilities are and how
they operate in the meaning-making activity we call language. This leads
to a different understanding of what a theoretical model should look like.
For example, the cognitive linguistic approach takes a view of the role of
theoretical economy that diverges greatly from that of Cartesian linguistics. The cognitive linguistic approach does not call for a new, language-
specific cognitive ability until it can be demonstrated that more general
abilities are insufficient to account for some aspect of linguistic behavior; and no such need has arisen yet in cognitive accounts of the range of
language abilities.

According to the cognitive linguistic view, biology is a better model
for understanding how language works than is formal logic or mechanis-
tic metaphors. Language abilities, like other biological phenomena, are
considered to be inherently uneconomical and redundant—they are assumed to be built up from the range of precursors that were available to
the evolving human species. Language then, under the cognitive approach,
is not created by an algorithmic grammar module; instead, it is constructed
(invented) by human beings using their general cognitive endowment. All
grammar does is supply speakers with an "inventory of symbolic resources"
(Langacker, 1988: 5).

Croft and Cruse identify three major hypotheses that guide the cognitive linguistic approach to language (2004: 1):

- Language is not an autonomous cognitive faculty
- Grammar is conceptualization
- Knowledge of language emerges from language use

The first hypothesis suggests that knowledge of language is no different from knowledge in general. In studying language, linguists working within a cognitive linguistic approach necessarily are interested in all types of knowledge, including models of memory, perception, and attention; the organization of knowledge into categories, prototypes, frames, schemas; the organization of conceptual structure into domains and spaces; and the dynamic cognitive processing that occurs whenever humans use language, such as coding and construal operations, including selection, point of view, and figure-ground organization. Cognitive linguists claim that these knowledge structures are based on embodied archetypes resulting from our lived interactions with the world, such as:

- Conceptions of objects moving in three-dimensional space
- Conceptions of the energetic interactions of objects and the transfer of energy
- Conceptions of viewing scenes from certain perspectives or vantage points
- Conceptions of real-world effects on our bodies, such as force dynamics and barriers

One striking feature of the cognitive linguistic framework is the remarkable degree to which visual perception enters into accounts of grammar. This is one area where signed languages can offer new insight, by providing data on language in the visual domain that are complementary to spoken language data.

The second hypothesis recognizes that it is not just within the realm of semantics that a cognitive approach to language is relevant: all grammar is seen as essentially symbolic. The lexicon, morphology, and syntax form a continuum of symbolic elements that provide for the linguistic structuring and construal of conceptual content.

The third hypothesis makes the critical assumption that the categories and conceptual structures that make up grammar are derived from our conception of specific utterances, actual uses of language. In order to account for the grammar of a language, the cognitive linguistic approach demands that we understand how general cognitive processes of schematization, abstraction, and generalization work to build up a conceptual model of language.

What about syntax? In order to approach the question of the origin of syntax, one must first take a position on what constitutes syntax. In the Cartesian approach to the study of language, syntax, semantics, and lexicon are distinct. A fundamental tenet of generative grammar is that syntax is "independent of all other levels of linguistic description including semantics—and independent of all other aspects of cognition as well" (Tomasello, 1998: ix–x). Under this view, grammatical ability is stipulated as part of the human genetic endowment, distinct from other perceptual and cognitive abilities. As we noted in chapter 2, the generativist Jackendoff has suggested that there are limitations to the syntactocentrism of generative grammar when there is interest in creating evolutionary scenarios for the origin of language.

Cognitive linguistics takes a radically different view. A fundamental tenet of cognitive linguistics is that lexicon, morphology, and syntax form a continuum of symbolic structures—symbolic because they possess both a phonological and a semantic pole. Words are symbolic structures, but according to cognitive grammar, so, too, is syntax. Such fundamental areas as grammatical class (e.g. nouns vs. verbs vs. prepositions), case, and basic grammatical relations (subject, direct object, indirect object) are shown to have semantic import that derives from *conceptual archetypes* having a nonlinguistic origin: "pre-linguistic conceptions grounded in everyday experience" that "reflect our experience as mobile and sentient creatures and as manipulators of physical objects" (Langacker, 1991a: 285). Under the cognitive linguistic view, there is no need to genetically stipulate a syntactic ability or module in the brain. The human language ability is assumed to require nothing more than genetically specified perceptual, cognitive, and motoric abilities.

Naturally, these two approaches to language lead to different positions on the role of gesture and iconicity in the origin of language. For generative linguists, syntax could not have evolved out of simpler structures such as animal communication or human gestural systems. Consider Chomsky (1972: 70):

> When we ask what human language is, we find no striking
> similarity to animal communication systems. . . . The examples
> of animal communication that have been examined to date do
> share many of the properties of human gestural systems, and it
> might be reasonable to explore the possibility of direct connec-
> tion in this case. But human language, it appears, is based on
> entirely different principles.

The cognitive approach is compatible with a view that language—not just lexicon but also syntax—could have emerged out of animal communication and human (or protohuman) gestural systems such as those discussed earlier. It is here that Stokoe's notion of *semantic phonology* plays a critical role in linking language and gesture. Stokoe described semantic phonology this way (1991: 112):

> The usual way of conceiving of the structure of language is
> linear: First there are the sounds (phonology), these are put
> together to make the words and their classes (morphology), the

words in turn, are found to be of various classes, and these are used to form phrase structures (syntax), and finally, the phrase structures, after lexical replacement of their symbols, yield meaning (semantics). A semantic phonology ties the last step to the first, making a seamless circuit of this progression. The metaphor for semantic phonology that jumps to mind is the Möbius strip: the input is the output, with a twist.

Semantic phonology suggests that signs are archetypal examples of self-symbolization. Like the twist in the Möbius strip, the phonological pole of gestures and signs consists of *something that acts and its action*. That is, hands and their actions are iconic manifestations of the conceptual arche-types that are the prelinguistic source of grammatical structures. Hands are prototypical nouns, and their actions are prototypical verbs. A hand can act transitively on another hand, transmitting energy to the impacted object; or a hand can act intransitively, as when we trace the path of an object that has moved. Semantic phonology links not only gesture and syntax but also signed and spoken language. It suggests that visible gestures were from the begin-ning critical elements in the origins of sign language grammar.

Thus, contrary to the generativist position that while human gesture may be related to animal communication, neither is directly connected to human language, semantic phonology contends that visible actions lie at the origin of all human languages. Support for this claim comes from a variety of sources. The recent evidence for mirror neurons suggests that gestural signs likely played a role in the evolution of human language in general, or in the evolution of the human *capacity* for language. Rizzolatti and Arbib note that the "precursor of Broca's area was endowed before speech appearance with a mechanism for recognizing actions made by others" (1998: 190) and suggest that this finding supports gestural theory: "language in humans . . . evolved from a basic mechanism originally not related to communication: the capacity to recognize actions" (193).

It is worth noting here that Chomsky has recently returned to the ques-tion of the origin and evolution of the human capacity for language, specifi-cally the "faculty of language" (Hauser, Chomsky, & Fitch, 2002). He and his colleagues conclude that, in fact, animal communication systems may have much to tell us about the precursors and evolution of aspects of what they term the "faculty of language—broad sense," defined as: "an internal computation system [faculty of language—narrow sense or FLN] combined with at least two other organism-internal systems, which we call 'sensory-motor' and 'conceptual-intentional'" (1570–71). The narrow language fac-ulty (FLN) included within the FLB turns out to be "narrow syntax," or essentially recursion, the human ability to create a virtually infinite num-ber of sentences from a finite lexicon. While Hauser, Chomsky, and Fitch conclude that aspects of the FLB, including categorical perception, speech

perception and production, and perhaps even theory of mind have homologues in nonhuman primates and other vertebrates, the FLN probably does
not. They speculate further that if nonhuman homologues for recursion are
found, they will be found in components of behavior other than those supporting communication, for example, number quantification, navigation, or
the maintenance of social relations. The latter point they leave open for further empirical research, and they conclude by calling for increased research
efforts from a variety of disciplines to attack the issue.

From our perspective, this is a positive step by Chomsky, and we are
not surprised that he would continue to maintain the recursive ability at
the heart of generative grammar as the one human linguistic trait without
nonhuman precursors or homologues. We believe, however, that it may
be possible to devise an argument for the evolution of recursion that does
involve communication—communication through manual gesture. We
pointed out in chapter 2 that Stokoe's notion of semantic phonology suggests that communication involving iconic manual gesture is inherently
recursive, and we will devote much of the rest of this book to working out
the consequences of that insight.

It is also worth noting that the psychologist David Premack has provided a follow-on to the argument developed by Hauser, Chomsky, and
Fitch. Commenting on work by Fitch and Hauser (2004) that finds a lack
of evidence of recursive grammatical ability in tamarin monkeys, Premack
outlines what he calls five "faculties that underlie the evolution of language" (2004: 319) and compares them among humans, chimpanzees, and
monkeys. With regard to his first faculty, voluntary control of the voice,
face, and hands, he concludes that only humans control all three but that
chimpanzees and monkeys control their hands. His second faculty is imi-
tation of instrumental action, and he says that humans and chimpanzees
possess it but that chimpanzees require human training to achieve it. The
third faculty, teaching, is said to be practiced only by humans, and his
fourth faculty, theory of mind, is posited in its recursive form only in humans but in chimpanzees in nonrecursive form. Finally, he discusses the
capacity to acquire recursive and nonrecursive grammar. With respect to
this fourth faculty, he finds that only humans are known to acquire both
kinds of grammar, but that chimpanzees and monkeys can acquire
nonrecursive grammar, while it has not yet been shown if they can also
acquire recursive grammar. Whether or not Premack is right about the status of these primates with respect to recursiveness, we want to reinforce
his point about the ancient origin of full voluntary control over the hands.

2.2 Theoretical Models and Language Evolution

The presuppositions and perspectives of these two approaches to language
have profound implications for what must be accounted for if language is

to emerge. For the Cartesian linguist, grammar is structure that exists independently from its use and from other cognitive abilities. In order to account for the emergence of language, the Cartesian must directly account for how grammar-as-structure emerged. It is little wonder that such a model leads to proposals that language emerged at once, in all its complexity: "syntax must have emerged in one piece, at one time—the most likely cause being some kind of mutation that affected the organization of the brain" (Bickerton, 1990: 190), or that the grammar organ evolved to serve some purpose other than communication (Hauser, Chomsky, & Fitch, 2002).

Although cognitive and functional linguists differ in some fundamental ways in their approach to the study of language, they share the view that grammar as structure is an emergent phenomenon. For the cognitive or the functional linguist, grammar emerges from use in social situations by individuals with general cognitive abilities. To account for the prehistoric emergence of language, cognitive and functional linguists need not account for how grammar emerged; instead, they must account for the presence of certain cognitive abilities, study their use in nonhuman primates, and hypothesize about the selection of these abilities in the hominid lineage.

Cognitive linguists are just now beginning to weigh in on the issue of the evolution of language. Fauconnier and Turner (2002), for example, devote a chapter to exploring the role that certain cognitive abilities might play in the emergence of language. One such ability, they suggest, is the construction of mental space blends.

Mental spaces are cognitive structures. Thinking relies on the construction and manipulation of mental spaces. In communicating, the words uttered by our interlocutor prompt us to construct mental spaces. For example, when we hear someone say *Tom bought a new computer,* we construct a simple mental space to account for this situation. Other mental spaces can be much more complex, such as those inviting us to construct mental spaces not only for a presupposed reality but also for an imagined situation counter to this reality, as when we say *If I was your father I'd spank you!*

Finally, mental spaces can be blended. Blends combine two or more mental spaces into a third "blended space," which uses features from both of the input mental spaces, but goes beyond each in important ways, too. A blended space is thus both less than and more than the sum of its parts. One example of a blended space described by Fauconnier (1997) is the "boat-race example." The example comes from a description of a "race" in which the modern-day catamaran *Great America II* sails from San Francisco to Boston in 1993. It follows the route of a clipper, the *Northern Light,* which did the same run in 1853. A few days before the *Great America II* reached Boston harbor, it would be possible to say:

At this point, *Great America II* is barely maintaining a 4.5-day
lead over *Northern Light*.

Obviously, *Northern Light* is not currently present, and *Great America II*
cannot possibly be running "ahead" of the clipper. What allows us to say
and to understand this sentence is that we can construct a blend that com-
bines the 1853 temporal space and the 1993 temporal space along with a
'race' mental space. The blend also creates an emergent structure not a part
of either of the input spaces in which the two ships are imagined to be trav-
eling on the same path at the same time, and so we can speak of the *Great
America II* as being "in the lead." As Fauconnier points out, blends create
not only novel expressions as in this example; they pervade human thought
and lead to the creation of novel ideas, new ways of seeing and understanding things, new insights and innovations.

Of course, our discussion of mental spaces and blends has taken place
in the context of linguistic communication. The important point, though,
is that there are complex cognitive processes going on that predate, underlie, and lead to linguistic outcomes. Our proposal is that the best way
to understand the development of these prerequisite cognitive abilities that
led to the emergence of language is to put *all of language* in the mix, spoken and signed. When we do this, we are led to how gestural theories of
language origins might be integrated with Fauconnier and Turner's proposal that the ability to construct mental space blends played a critical role
in the emergence of language. And this in turn yields a more encompass-
ing cognitive view of language evolution.

Questions that might be addressed include:

- What role did hand actions play in the evolution of language?
  Fauconnier and Turner (2002: 376) point out the importance of
  human-scale constructions for space, force, and motion in the
  development of the cognitive ability to perform blends. They go
  on to say that "human action, with motion and intentionality in
  physical space and time, is a basic human-scale structure" (378).
  Does the close link between manual activity and language suggest
  that intentionally moving the hand was a critical human action
  that fostered the cognitive abilities that would eventually underlie the language ability?
- Even the casual reader of cognitive linguistics cannot help but be
  struck by the pervasive use of visual perception in accounting for
  the cognitive abilities that underlie human language, especially
  construal operations so important to grammar. One may wonder
  whether this is merely an expository device, or whether in fact
  visual perceptual abilities are central to language. If they are,

what does this suggest for the role of visible actions in the
emergence of language?
- Might semantic phonology, as manifest through the pervasive
cognitive iconicity found in signed languages, be an archetypal
example of mental space blending?

Obviously the cognitive linguistic exploration of the evolution of language is just beginning. Even at this early stage, however, it is clear that
there are numerous ways in which the cognitive linguistic study of gesture and signed languages can inform a new approach to the study of the
evolution of language.

3 Ritualization and Cognition:
Grounding Language in the Body

According to the perspective we are developing, three critical elements are
implicated in the evolution of language: cognitive abilities, the process of
ritualization, and visible gesture. It is tempting to regard cognitive abilities
as essential to the individual and ritualization as a social process, but this
would be a misleading dichotomy. Among the primates, cognitive abilities
surely evolve within the context of social life, and the ritualization process
depends on the presence of certain preexisting cognitive abilities. Nevertheless, the cognitive abilities we are concerned with here are abilities that
individuals bring to bear on their perceptual and motoric interactions with
the world, whether physical or social.

Ritualization critically involves repetition. A ritualized activity need
not ever occur in a social situation. One might develop a completely private
ritual to follow when one is shaving, for example—no one would affect or
be affected by this ritual. Clearly, when we regard ritualization in this way,
it is not independent of cognitive abilities such as automaticization; however, it could also have a significant social impact. Conventionalization, a
process critical to language, is clearly a related phenomenon, a type of socially agreed-on ritual.

Visible gesture is a critical raw material on which cognitive abilities
and the process of ritualization may act in the creation of language. It plays
a mediating role in this creative process, providing, at different levels and
stages of development, various semiotic potentials on which natural selection could act. According to this model, gestures range from the articu-
lations made during the production of spoken (phonetic gestures, which
are not, for the most part, visible) or signed language to nonsymbolic actions that serve only instrumental and not communicative functions.

In cognitive linguistics, language is analyzed as a structured inventory of conventional linguistic units (Langacker, 1987). Cognitive linguis-

tics imposes a content requirement on linguistic units: "The only units permitted in the grammar of a language are (i) semantic, phonological, and symbolic structures that occur overtly in linguistic expressions; (ii) structures that are schematic for those in (i); and (iii) categorizing relationships involving the structures (i) and (ii)" (Langacker, 1991b: 18–19). Thus, the content requirement directly addresses one of the assumptions of the Cartesian approach—the grounding of language by ruling out all the arbitrary descriptive devices needed to support the formal machinery of a hypothesized autonomous syntactic module. These would include the surface and deep structures, rewrite rules, derivational trees, X-bar structures, and so on of evolving Chomskyan linguistics.

Cognitive linguistics claims that grammar (that is, syntax) is intrinsically symbolic. By using the term "symbolic," cognitive linguists do not mean that grammar can be described in terms of symbols that are manipulated by a set of rules that make no reference to the meanings of the symbols, as in Chomskyan generative grammar. Instead, the term "symbol" refers to a unit that has both phonological and semantic substance. Although symbolic units may exist at various levels of abstraction, they are restricted to structures that possess both form and meaning, unlike the abstract syntax of generative grammar that possesses form only. Symbolic units in the sense of cognitive linguistics are the building blocks of grammar—grammar is nothing but highly schematized symbolic units. It is for this reason that cognitive linguists claim that lexicon, morphology, and syntax form a continuum of symbolic structures (Langacker, 1988).

A basic claim of cognitive linguistics is that grammatical constructions embody conventional imagery, where imagery is taken to mean the ability to mentally construe a situation in alternate ways. The cognitive linguistic approach depends on a number of basic cognitive abilities to account for the functioning of grammar:

1. The ability to form structured conceptualizations.
2. The ability to establish correspondences between components of different conceptualizations.
3. Entrenchment (also called routinization, automaticization, and habituation). This is the process in which, through repetition, a complex structure comes to be manipulable as a prepackaged assembly. It is through entrenchment that a complex structure becomes manipulable as a unit; the unit becomes reified.
4. Abstraction, or the emergence of structure through reinforcement of the commonality inherent in multiple experiences.
5. Schematization, a special case of abstraction in which a coarse-grained commonality emerges when distinct structures are viewed with less precision and specificity (from a distant vantage point). A schema is the commonality that emerges from

distinct structures when one abstracts away from their points of
difference by portraying them with less precision and specificity.

6. Comparison, or the ability to detect differences between two (or
more) structures. Comparison involves an inherent asymmetry
whereby one structure serves as a standard against which a
target is evaluated.

7. Categorization. This is a type of comparison in which the
standard is an established unit and the target is originally novel.
When there is no discrepancy, the target provides more information about the standard; when there is, the target extends the
standard.

8. Composition, or the ability to combine simpler structures into
more complex ones. Composition involves the ability to
integrate two or more component structures to form a composite
structure.

9. Association, or the process in which one kind of experience
evokes another.

10. Symbolization, which is a particular kind of association in
which conceptualizations are associated with observable
entities such as sounds, visible gestures, or written marks.

11. The ability to impose figure-ground organization on a scene.
That is, scenes do not come with "objective" figure-ground
organization; instead, this organization is a matter of construal.
Describing a situation as "the couch is under the picture" or
"the picture is above the couch" imposes figure-ground organization on an objective scene.

12. Focusing (profiling). This is the ability to select or focus
attention on one aspect of a complex scene (for example, the
ability to select a standard and a target).

13. The ability to track an entity though time. This cognitive ability
depends on perceptual continuity.

The way cognitive linguistics uses cognitive abilities like these to account for grammatical phenomena is beyond the scope of this discussion.
However, we would like to make a few observations about this list of abilities. First, they have a deep association with spatial abilities. The connections between language ability and spatial cognition are also explored by
another branch of cognitive linguistics that deals with "mental spaces"
(Fauconnier, 1995; Fauconnier & Turner, 1996). It is worth noting that linguists of signed languages are increasingly making use of this work (e.g.
Liddell, 2003). Deane presents a unified theory of syntax consistent with
the tenets of cognitive linguistics; he provides compelling linguistic evidence and neurological data from the study of aphasia to support his claim
that that there is a "close connection between bodily experience, spatial

thought and grammar" (1992: 4). The evolutionary role of spatial cognition is clearly an important part of the story of the emergence of language.

Second, these cognitive abilities also have a close connection with vision and visual cognition. This is clear with respect to not only those abilities that are explicitly based in vision, such as imagery, focus, and figure-ground organization, but also such basic cognitive abilities as schematization and categorization. This link between vision and language has been noted by others as well. For example, the cognitive scientist Martin Sereno (1991a, 1991b) claims that language may well have emerged from a fairly simple modification of visual cognition. He notes analogies between "scene perception" and language:

> The integration of successive glances in the comprehension of a visual scene requires a kind of serial assembly operation similar in some respects to the integration of word meanings in discourse comprehension. . . . The underspecified, context-free information in an isolated glance is sharpened and focused by context (cf. polysemy); information from temporally distant glances must be tied together (cf. anaphora). (1991a: 82)

The main difference between scene perception and language, according to Sereno, is that comprehending a scene is closely tied to the current scene, whereas language "might best be thought of as a kind of fictive visual scene comprehension, in the case of spoken language comprehension, by sequences of phoneme[s]" (Sereno, 1991b: 82).

The difference is less stark, however, when we broaden our view to include language or communicative behavior that is not spoken. Here we see an example of how visible gestures play a mediating role in the path from vision to voice. If we imagine a case in which a story is presented primarily by means of visible gestures, we see immediately that visible gestures are both a part of the current visual scene and about some fictive (or remembered or hypothetical) scene. Moreover, the inherently cinematic, in the sense of scene-oriented, nature of poetry and storytelling in ASL has recently been explored by Bauman (2003).

The linguist Talmy Givón has developed a theoretical framework for language evolution that is in many ways compatible with what we are presenting here. He suggests that language arose "through co-evolution of the neuro-cognitive mechanisms, socio-cultural organization and communicative skills of pre-human hominids" (1995: 444). A central thesis of his proposal is that the neurological underpinnings of human language processing are an evolutionary consequence of the *"visual information processing system"* (394). Givón notes that the visual processing system splits into two streams in the brain: a ventral visual processing stream that analyzes visually perceived objects as belonging to particular types, and a dorsal stream that is responsible for analyzing spatial relations and spatial motions among specific objects. He identifies correspondences between these two streams and linguistic processing: (1) Recognizing an object as a member of a generic type is the visual equivalent of lexical-semantic identification, which involves recognizing a specific token of a word as an exemplar of a generic type, and (2) recognizing spatial relations among objects, or between an object figure and its spatial ground, is the equivalent of recognizing propositional information about states or events, because propositions are about relationships (408–409).

A third generalization about human cognitive abilities is that there is a strong manipulative component to many of them. It is no accident that in many languages, people resort to words that originate as descriptions of manipulative behavior to describe certain cognitive abilities. In English, when we have understood an idea, when we have finally come to grips with it, we have *grasped* it. As we stress throughout this book, all of these cognitive abilities are ultimately traceable to the way of life of the ancestral higher primates—they were arboreal creatures whose master sensory system was vision and whose lives depended on the ability to accurately grasp small objects.

We can sum this up by noting that the cognitive abilities we have discussed here, which are the foundation for the human language capacity, are grounded in the visual perception and manipulation of objects and events in the world. While this conclusion is compatible with the cognitive linguistic view of human language, it is exactly contrary to a critical claim of Cartesian linguistics—that language is a disembodied symbolic property of the human mind and that it is not grounded in peripheral (perceptual and motoric) systems.

3.1 Ritualization

Haiman (1994, 1998b) presents the most compelling case for the role of ritualization in the evolution of language. He points out that the driving force in ritualization is repetition of a specific behavior. He identifies three major processes associated with ritualization: *emancipation*, or the freeing of instrumental actions from their primary motivation; *habituation*, or a decline in the strength of response or even the tendency to respond to a repeated stimulus; and *automaticization*. Berger and Luckman defined automaticization by observing that "any action that is repeated frequently becomes cast into a pattern, which can then be reproduced with an economy of effort" (1966: 53).

All three processes are at work across human and nonhuman behaviors and across linguistic and nonlinguistic behaviors. The first, emancipation, plays a key role in semanticization, the transformation of an instrumental act into a sign. Automaticization is responsible for the emergence of double articulation (duality of patterning), which many regard as a hallmark of human language. Habituation brings about the transformation of icons into arbitrary symbols, signs that are not motivated by their links to external referents and that are therefore susceptible to systemic or internal constraints on their forms. We will discuss these processes in greater depth later.

4 Visible Gesture: Making Meaning with Motion

It is useful to consider the various types of gestures that can be produced and received by animals. We might consider which parts of the animal's body can be engaged in the production of gestures and thus unavailable for other activities or, conversely, which activities preclude the production of gestures. For example, in chapter 2 we pointed to the fundamental importance of the evolution of bipedalism in freeing the hands for manual gesturing—it is very difficult to produce a manual gesture while engaged in an activity, such as quadrupedal locomotion, that requires the use of both hands.

We might also consider how the receiving animal perceives the sender's gesture—or, more correctly, how it perceives the proximal signal (optic or acoustic in the case of an emerging capacity for language)—produced by the distal gestural organ—as well as the physical properties of the signal. Optical gestures require a visual system and a source of light for perception—visible gestures are less efficient in the dark and in environments that block vision (e.g., arboreal environments when the communicating animals are at a distance from each other). Visible gestures also require that the sending animal be in the visual field of the receiver, optimally at the center of the receiver's visual attention. It is also true that we cannot optimally receive more than one visual signal at a time, because we can only attend to one. Other sources of visual information that might be available in the environment become less accessible or even inaccessible to an animal that needs to attend to a stream of visible gestures.

Acoustic signals have a different set of characteristics. The ear does not have to be directed at the signaling source in order to receive an acoustic signal—these signals are equally effective in the dark as in the light and are better suited to long-range communication in arboreal environments than are optical signals. Ears have no other function (except as occasional vehicles for decoration in some human societies) than to receive acoustic signals. Although auditory attention can certainly be directed ("Children, pay attention to me!"), it is also true that we can perceive auditory information to which we are not attuned—consider the common experience of overhearing your name being spoken while you are engaged in another conversation. Acoustic information is complementary to optical information.

Some of these characteristics, as we have already suggested in chapter 2 and as we will discuss more fully later, make linguistic communication in the acoustic medium advantageous. However, as we argue throughout this book, the crucial step from gesture to language must have occurred in the optical gestural medium. This is true because at the early stages of the emergence of language, it is visible gestures that mediate action and communication. Visible gestures are at once actions in the world, actions with instrumental function (grasping prey), and, at least potentially, communicative actions, acts that convey information, intent, and relationship ("I grasped the prey"). It is not merely that visible gestures can be iconic for objects and events in the world—visible gestures *are* objects and events in the world.

5 Ritualization: Semanticization and Grammaticization

Ritualization plays two critical roles in this evolutionary framework. First, it is implicated in the initial emergence of communication, a process that can be equated with the sociobiological notion of semanticization: "In the course of evolution, both locomotory movements and acts (concerned with comfort, with heat regulation, and with the capture of prey) have been selected and modified to produce signals" (Blest, 1963: 102). Givón describes the process of semanticization as a transformation of instrumental behavior into communicative signals. He claims that this process can be broken down into several distinct components (1995, 429):

1. A complex, thick band of co-occurring features of behavior co-occurs reliably with a unique referent.
2. Attention is gradually narrowed from the entire thick band to a few or one of its salient features.
3. The single salient feature is then reinterpreted as a communicative clue.
4. All other features of the behavior are disregarded.

Second, ritualization is involved in the transformation of these primitive signals into grammaticalized signs—signs with features that we regard as criteria of human language, such as double articulation (duality of patterning), arbitrariness, and digitization. Thus, ritualization is implicated in the emergence of communicative signaling and in the transformation of nonlinguistic signals into linguistic signs.

Semanticization is driven by the first of the three types of ritualization mentioned earlier, emancipation. Emancipation refers to the transformation of objects and events in the world into signs; that is, objects or events that stand for something else, especially for categories of things.

As behaviors are emancipated from their instrumental functions, they can be selected and modified to act as signals. Acts that formerly served instrumental functions become free to take on meaning. Haiman cites a paradigmatic example from research on the mating activity of balloon, or dancing, flies. The male balloon fly signals the female that he is available for mating by giving her a "wedding present"—a balloon-like object made of silk that he produces. He does this, apparently to distract the female, who would just as soon eat the male as mate with him. While she is busy opening the present, he mounts and mates with her. According to Haiman, this is the explanation for the male's ritualized gesture (1994: 4):

> Originally, the male dancing fly distracted the predaceous female
> with a distracting gift of a dead insect: at this point, the gift was
> purely instrumental. Later, the gift was interpreted as a signal to
> the female, a signal whose message was something like "this fly
> is available for mating." Originally, also, the male partially
> wrapped his tiny prey up in silk exuded from his anal glands,
> probably in order to subdue it: the silk, like the dead insect, had
> an instrumental function, and its similarity to "wrapping" was
> incidental. Finally, however, the mate achieved his original
> "purpose" by giving the female the elaborated wrapping alone,
> and it is the wrapping which serves as the mating signal.

Thus, in the nonlinguistic realm, instrumental actions—movements or gestures—are ritualized through repetition and become meaningful acts—signals. These basic, paradigmatic cases of semanticization invariably involve the transformation of instrumental, visible gestures into meaningful signals.

Haiman also suggests that emancipation transforms connotation into denotation—that denotation is emancipated connotation. The process operates like this (1998b: 153):

> A symptomatic gesture or fidget (let us say a cry of pain like
> [aaaa]) accompanies a psychological state. That is, originally
> the gesture co-occurs with the state. It becomes a signal which
> connotes that state once it is recognized and responded to by
> some other animal. Finally, it becomes a sign (say, the English
> word "ouch") which denotes the state only when it becomes
> emancipated both from the stimulus which produced it origi-

nally and from the motivated state of which it served as a
signal.

It was at this early stage of semanticization, which Haiman regards as
marking the true origin of language, that visible gestures played a key role,
because they can resemble physically what they mean. In this regard, they
exhibit what Peirce (1955) called *image iconicity*. But more is required to
get to language. It is one thing to account for the emergence of meaningful
signs—signs that can iconically represent objects, actions, and events in
the world. It is quite another matter to account for linguistic signs, which
do more than name—they also enter into relations with other signs and
thereby represent relationships among objects, actions, and events in the
world. Iconic visible gestures, as we have shown in our discussion of semantic phonology, go beyond simply representing events and actions—
they also carry the seed of syntax—they are both name and relation. As
such, they exhibit a second type of iconicity, *diagrammatic iconicity*—the
relations among parts of the sign correspond to or reflect relations among
parts of what they refer to (Peirce, 1955).

The diagrammatic iconicity of visible gestures is both externally and
internally directed. Visible, particularly manual, gestures not only iconically represent the structures of events but also stand in an iconic relationship to the internal structure of linguistic signs. Events in the world can
be construed as involving objects and interactions. Objects are prototypi-
cally stable through time and are capable of moving about and interacting
with other objects. Objects are conceptually autonomous with respect to
interactions. These characteristics and values map onto linguistic signs,
which not only represent objects and interactions in the world but also
consist of prototypical objects (nouns) and interactions (verbs) with their
own patterns of relationship.

The same characteristics apply to visible gestures: They are diagrammatically iconic with syntactic relations. They are objects that move about
and interact with other objects. Hands are prototypical nouns, and their
actions are prototypical verbs. Hands, as objects, are conceptually autonomous with respect to the interactions they can enter into (grabbing, pull-
ing, tearing, hitting, etc.). The production and perception of visible, manual
gestures ground grammar in action and perception. Archetypal semantic
roles such as agent and patient, and archetypal events such as transitive
actions, are grounded in our visual perception of manual gestures and our
experience as mobile manipulators of objects. We will explore these notions further in chapter 5, where we discuss cognitive iconicity.

In summary, it was this nexus of functions and correspondences that
made visible gesture the key element in the emergence of language. Visible gesture, like the Roman god Janus, faces in two directions simultaneously: toward the perceived world of objects and events and toward the

conceived world of grammar. Visible gestures are: (1) instrumental actions in the world; (2) potentially communicative actions about the world; (3) diagrammatically iconic with objects and events in the world; and (4) diagrammatically iconic with syntactic relations.

Semanticization provides a mechanism by which we can get from instrumental gestures to meaningful gestures—that is, primitive linguistic signs. But two problems remain. First, if visible gesture was so critical to the emergence of language, then why is language not now generally based on visible signs? Kendon (1991: 215) also posed this question: "All forms of language that we encounter today (with the exception of the relatively rare occurrence of primary, i.e. deaf sign languages, and the even rarer development of alternative sign languages in speaking communities) are, of course, spoken. If language began as gesture, why did it not stay that way?" In an earlier work, one of us (Wilcox, 2004b) called this the "Great Switch" from visible gesture to speech. How can our framework account for this?

The second problem concerns what happened after the switch. If, in the switch to speech, we find a sudden appearance of those critical features of language such as arbitrariness, double articulation, and digitization, then we have in fact explained very little. How do we account for the appearance of grammaticalized speech from a visible gestural precursor?

6 From Vision to Voice

We believe that the same cognitive abilities, ritualization processes, and characteristics of visible gesture that were used to account for the emergence of the first linguistic gestures can also be used to account for the transition to speech and the appearance of the features that we now consider to be characteristic of modern spoken languages.

First, we claim here (as we have elsewhere in Armstrong, Stokoe, & Wilcox, 1995: 42) that there was in fact no Great Switch from gesture to speech. One answer to Kendon's question is that speech is still gestural. The difference between visible gestures and speech sounds is not that one is gestural and other is not—they are both gestural in the sense that both depend on planned sequences of musculo-skeletal actions. The operative difference is that one is visible/optical and the other is audible/acoustic. But this begs Kendon's question to some extent.

The unique semiotic qualities of visible gestures as both actions-in-the-world and communicative actions were critical in moving from action to meaning—in semanticizing visible actions. But these visible gestures did not occur alone; our ancestors were not mute, as we noted in chapter 2. Remember that in an arboreal environment, vocal communication will be vastly more useful for distance communication than will be visible gesture. Visible gesture and audible gesture were surely both present in a rich, holistic, action-communication system. Once visible gestures became emancipated from their instrumental functions and became primitive signs within this complex visible-audible gestural system, the same process of emancipation came to bear on this new system. Only now, audible gestures came to be symptomatic for the visible-audible gestural complex. Here is how this process maps onto the steps involved in emancipation that we considered earlier:

1. "A complex thick band of co-occurring features of behavior co-occurs reliably with a unique referent": *Visible gesture and audible gesture co-occur as a complex, multimodal signal.*
2. "Attention is gradually narrowed from the entire thick band to a few or one of its salient features": *Attention is redirected from the multimodal signal to the acoustic portion of it.*
3. "The single salient feature is then reinterpreted as a communicative clue": *Audible gesture is construed as representing the entire signal.*
4. "All other features of the behavior are disregarded": *The visible gestural portion of the complex signal decreases in communicative salience and is able to serve other functions.*

In other words, a sudden shift from gesture to speech never occurred. In this scenario, there never was a time when visible gestures were unaccompanied by vocalizations, and there has never been a time when speech was unaccompanied by visible gestures, as it still is today. Instead, there was a gradual realignment of information transmission during which the primary load of linguistic information shifted from the visible to the acoustic.

This scenario has the added advantage of accounting for the deep neurological and psychological linkages between speech and visible gesture that have been noted by several researchers (e.g. Blake, 2000; Kimura, 1993; McNeill, 1992). According to our scenario, they have always existed as interlinked parts of a complex system. As we have already noted, Cartesian linguistics has historically posited a possible connection between animal communication and human gesture but no connection between animal communication and human language—according to Chomsky (1972: 70), they are based on entirely different principles. How then do we explain the linkage between human gesture and speech? Although the most dogmatic statement of the Cartesian position may be starting to erode even with respect to Chomsky himself (Hauser, Chomsky, & Fitch, 2002), we think our scenario provides the most parsimonious explanation.

What might have caused the realignment in the roles of visible gesture and vocalization within this evolving system? We indicated some of the more simple-minded possible explanations in chapter 3: speech may be more energy efficient than signing, speech frees the hands for tool use and for demonstration of other manual techniques to novices, speech is effective in the dark and past opaque obstacles, hearing does not require directed attention as does vision. Here we will attempt to integrate these ideas into a somewhat more comprehensive account utilizing King's (1994) notion of social information "donation" among primates. King's model explains how and why increased information donation was selected for: "The clearest pattern for information donation is found in the foraging context and correlates with food sharing and extractive foraging with tools" (117). King claims that "a likely selection pressure for greater donation of information is a shift to dependence on foods that require a significant investment by immatures in acquiring foraging skills and the information on which those skills depend" (119).

Acquisition of foraging and tool-making skills relies critically on at least two processes. First, adult and immature animals must jointly attend to the task at hand. This means cognitively sharing a focus on, say, digging up a tuber in a certain way or producing a tool with a certain technique, as well as visually attending to the task. As tasks become increasingly complex, the demand for information donation to take place through explicit instruction will also become greater. This is precisely where the use of visible gestures would place foragers and learners at a disadvantage. Visible gestures require the hands, which are engaged in another activity, and the eyes, which must divide their attention between attending to the task and attending to the gesturer. Obviously, this would favor shifting emphasis to the acoustic channel to carry at least part of the communicative load, simultaneously relieving the optical channel for the receipt of other important information. The same case can be made for information donation related to other complex tasks, where selection would sometimes favor the optical channel and other times the acoustic. The important point here is that the same ritualization processes that accounted for the transformation of instrumental visible activities into complex meaningful gestures could also account for the realignment of a visible-audible gestural complex in which visible gestures initially carried the bulk of the information load into a system in which audible gestures came to predominate.

7 Linguistic Ritualization: From Vocalizations to Phonemes

Burling (1993) suggests that of the many features of human language, the most important may be the principle of contrast. The principle of contrast is closely related to another feature of language, digitization: "The phonological system of a language, by imposing absolute distinctions on the phonetic continuum, is almost pure contrast, but we can also speak of words and even sentences as being in contrast. . . . The result is a digital system of communication constructed from contrasting signals" (28). As many have observed, this system of contrast at the sublexical level when combined with the rules of syntax makes possible the creation of an infinite number of meaningful expressions using a finite and strictly limited set of basic elements. Animal communication, on the other hand, is supposed to consist of a set of potentially continuously varying unitary expressions that have the capacity to convey information about a strictly limited set of possible events or states. Fundamentally, according to this view, human language is digital and animal communication is analog. As we noted earlier, human gesture in this view is also analog, and it probably has an evolutionary relationship with animal communication. For example, if we apply heat to a nonhuman primate, the loudness of its scream is likely to vary with the amount of heat we apply. If we do the same to a human, we might get the same result, or, depending on the level of our victim's sang-froid, we might get something like this: "On a scale of one to ten, that's a ten!" Or a nine, an eight, and so on.

Features other than contrast have also been noted as separating language from other forms of communication. Among the most commonly offered examples are duality of patterning (also known as double articulation) and arbitrariness (e.g., Hockett, 1982). One concern for those attempting to account for the evolution of language is to locate these features (or plausible precursors) in nonlinguistic animal communication or else to explain how they could have emerged from earlier communication systems that did not involve signs with arbitrary associations with their referents, were not pervasively contrastive (that is, had signals that varied continuously), and did not display duality of patterning. Haiman (1994, 1998b) provides an answer: these features are all emergent properties of language, the artifacts of ritualization.

Let us first consider the principles of contrast and digitization. As we saw earlier, emancipation is implicated in the transformation of instrumental action into signals. Emancipation is also implicated in the further transformation of these signals—it is involved in codification, or the creation of signs. Codification operates on actions in two ways. First, the activity, through ritualization, becomes routinized—its form remains relatively stable, independent of the stimulus. Second, the routinized activity becomes decontextualized. Because it is not dependent for its expression on the presence of the initial stimulus, it can now occur in a variety of contexts. One result of codification in an emerging linguistic system is that what were originally random fluctuations become both distinctive and uniform, precisely because they were emancipated from their conditioning environments (see Haiman, 1994).

Digitization also results from the process by which signals become distinctive and uniform. Another way to characterize the process is to say that it is an example of what ethologists have called "typical intensity," or the tendency for a ritualized gesture to remain constant regardless of the presence or strength of the stimulus that produced it. The close connection between typical intensity in ritualized animal behavior and the properties of digitization and contrast in human language is revealed in the following observation from Blest (1963: 104): "Whereas stimuli of varying strength for the release of the unritualized precursors of display movements elicit responses of varying intensity and form, following ritualization, the derived responses acquire an almost constant form and intensity to a wide range of stimulus strengths."

Thus, when applied to the emergence of linguistic behavior, ritualization has two results. First, it can explain how previously variable or analog signals can become digital, so that linguistic units—phonemes, for example—impose absolute distinctions. Second, these emerging linguistic units can begin to form a system and thus enter into intrasystemic relations; that is, they become contrastive.

What about duality of patterning? This term refers to the structural organization of language at two levels that are deemed to be governed by independent sets of rules—the rules for assembling the meaningless units (phonemes) into meaningful units (morphemes) and the rules for assembling the morphemes into words and sentences. But meaningless units don't have to start that way—as we have already seen with respect to semantic phonology in signed languages, the process that drives duality of patterning is the erosion of meaningful units into meaningless units, and the same process is at work in the emergence of speech. This process is also identified with grammaticization, the erosion of meaning or substance through repeated use (Bybee, Perkins, & Pagliuca, 1994). Grammaticization as an organizing principle here is particularly important, because it leads to the erosion of larger units into smaller ones. Moreover, Haiman (1994: 111) suggests that we look at double articulation in a larger context, not simply as the separation between the meaningless and the meaningful in language but in terms of a hierarchy of larger to smaller units of organization. We have reproduced his scheme as figure 4.1.

There is clear cross-linguistic evidence that this grammaticization process, by which lexical expressions are reduced and lose semanticity, is pervasive and unidirectional (Bybee et al., 1994). What is clear also is that this process very much resembles ritualization, and it can be traced backward through time to include the ritualization of instrumental, nonlinguistic gestures—that is, it can account for the evolution of nonlanguage into language.

What about the arbitrariness of the sign—explicitly considered one of the hallmarks of human language since at least Shakespeare (a rose by any

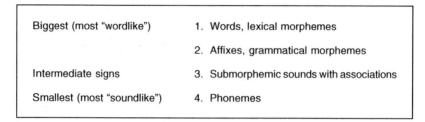

Figure 4.1. Hierarchy of double articulation. After John Haiman, "Ritualization and the Development of Language," in W. Pagliuca (ed.), *Perspectives on Grammaticalization* (Amsterdam: John Benjamins), 111.

other name). Certainly, the roots of arbitrariness are also revealed by many of the facets of ritualization just described. First, we saw that one result of ritualization is the emancipation of a signal from its motivation—the form loses its proximal motivation. Second, the beginnings of arbitrariness are also implied in the emergence of typical intensity. Manning (1967: 138) has elaborated on this theme: "Postures or movements which have a typical intensity are more easily recognized but correspondingly convey less information about the signaler's motivational state" (1967: 138). As the signal conveys less and less information about the motivation of the particular form of behavior, that form becomes more arbitrary in relation to what is being signified.

Finally, arbitrariness has its beginnings in another result of ritualization, the tendency for the form of the ritualized activity to become stylized. Stylized gestures or signals have hypertrophied to the point that they are instrumentally dysfunctional—the male balloon fly's offering to the female no longer contains food. Once emancipated from their functional motivation, they are free to take on a life of their own. We see two results that, at first glance, appear contradictory.

First, we see the rise of style for style's sake—increased sensitivity to system-internal constraints, as opposed to those that are system-external (motivated or iconic). Freed from practical, functional demands, stylization runs riot. Cartmill (1993) describes a telling example. Among the fourteenth-century English aristocracy, hunting was no longer a necessary activity. Freed from its role as a necessary food-producing activity, hunting became ritualized, stylized, and thus associated with upper-class status and gentility. Being familiar with the obligations of style, as a means of solidifying one's identity as a member of the gentry, became so important that aristocrats spent a great deal of time and effort learning proper hunting behavior: "The growth of ritual in the upper-class medieval hunt is documented in the how-to books produced for the education and training of aristocratic hunters. . . . [These books] became progressively more concerned with the forms of hunting etiquette and ceremony than with the practical task of bagging game" (61–62). The well-heeled medieval hunter had to learn a vast terminology for the various kinds of animal droppings, for the common configurations of antlers, for the hoofprints of deer, for the places where deer left signs of having lain or stood or walked or galloped, and for the different kinds of hunting dogs and their anatomy, behavior and so forth (64). Classical education has served a similar function, although an old adage reveals the extent to which ritualization may replace instrumental function with form: "It is not necessary actually to know Latin, it is sufficient merely to have forgotten it." The function of all of this in boundary maintenance between social classes reminds us also of the similar function of language registers—the more difficult a particular register is to master, the more effective it is at protecting the boundary, as Eliza Doolittle discovered and as Bill Cosby is currently reminding young African Americans.

Second, stylization leads to the development of standardization. Freed from external and idiosyncratic motivations or stimuli, activities, gestures, and signals become uniform. When stylization is applied to material culture, such as the production of tools and art objects, it places increased demands on explicit instruction and thus on information donation (King, 1994: 102–109). In human languages, these properties are manifested in the following ways: standardization implies internal structure or standards of well-formedness—that is, grammar; and, since these standards have only internal coherence and little, if any, external motivation (they represent "grammar for grammar's sake"), the only way they can persist is through convention.

Using ritualization in a scenario for language evolution has one significant benefit that is lacking in other accounts of what distinguishes language from nonlanguage—it suggests a mechanism driving the emergence of the distinguishing features of language. For example, Burling (1993, 1999) builds the case that human language (or language-like) systems are sharply separated from the human gesture-call system (and from animal gesture-call systems), in the mode of Chomsky. However, he does not offer an explanation for how the features he believes are critical to language came to be, other than that they reflect some sort of general cognitive advancement for humans, rather than an advance in communication. Saying that "language emerged as a product of our evolving mind" (1993: 36) does not explain why language has the features of contrast and digitization, arbitrariness, and duality of patterning. Are these simply properties of an evolving mind and not an evolving communication system (as Chomsky seems to be continuing to maintain, even as he seriously considers the evolution of language for the first time—Hauser, Chomsky, & Fitch, 2002)?

While it seems inescapable that emerging cognitive abilities were significant in the emergence of language, we have to ask: which is the cart and which is the horse? While it is important to study how animals use their minds (even acknowledging that animals might have minds is a step forward), we must also recognize that minds are emergent properties of social life (Mead, 1970; Vygotsky, 1978). Because of this, we cannot extricate the mind from communication. Minds did not emerge in individuals living in isolation; they emerged in individuals who were participants in social units and among whom communication was taking place.

8 The Emergence of Grammar: An Ongoing Process

One implication of the previous discussion is that there was no single event that occurred at a particular point in time (such as a genetic mutation or the sudden "discovery" of symbols or symbol traces) that we can identify as the point of origin of language. Evolution is not a process that happened only once, in the past—it goes on continually, and this is equally true of the evolution of language and grammar. Grammar is always emerging. We agree with Taylor (1996) that the origin of language never happened—it is always happening.

This is also the view of functional linguists such as Hopper (1998), who argue that grammar is an emergent property of language. But this view of language also suggests something more fundamental. Not only do the grammars of existing languages continue to emerge, but we might be able to watch this process as it occurs, if we look in the right place. Not surprisingly, we think that the right place to look is where language might be expected to arise as visible gesture.

We will consider the historical emergence of full-fledged signed languages in chapter 7, but a particularly instructive example comes from a study of the evolution of language on a microgenetic time scale. Singleton, Morford, and Goldin-Meadow (1993) present evidence that when individuals invent symbols to communicate de novo, they can generate a system that is characterized by what they call "internal standards of well-formedness." Their data come from two sources: gestures invented by a deaf child, David, over a period of years, and gestures invented by nonsigning hearing individuals on the spot.

This important study provides a glimpse at the emergence of language in action. Standards of well-formedness are defined as "the organization of information in contrastive and productive categories" (Singleton, Morford, & Goldin-Meadow, 1993: 705). The authors note that David's gestures displayed two features: they conveyed information about the referent of the gesture (that is, they were iconically motivated), and they fit into a contrastive system of form/meaning categories. The difference between gestures that conform to standards of well-formedness and those that do not is captured in the difference between gestures invented by novice gesturers for the first time and David's system of home-grown signs that he developed over extended periods of time by interacting with the hearing people around him (703–704):

> When the novice gesturers generated a gesture, their goal was to produce a handshape that adequately represented the object, and their choice of handshapes appeared to be constrained only by their imaginations and the physical limitations imposed by the hands themselves. In contrast, when David generated a gesture, his choice of handshape was (we suggest) guided not only by how well a handshape captured the features of an object, but also by how well that handshape fit into the set of handshapes allowed in his system.

The novice gesturers' creations were motivated. David's gestures, although still partially sensitive to external motivation (i.e., they were iconic), "conformed to an internally consistent and contrastive system; that is, they appeared to have standards of form" (710).

Our only quibble is with the ontological status of these standards of well-formedness, because clearly their manifestation in David's gestures amounts to the appearance of a grammar. Throughout their study, the authors seem to assume a Cartesian model of language: "In this paper, we explore the forces propelling a communication system toward standards of well-formedness" (Singleton, Morford, & Goldin-Meadow, 1993: 648). The authors imply that these standards are preexisting (presumably in David's mind) and that they direct the course of the emerging language system. The authors seem to be saying that David relied on an innate, mental representation of standards of well-formedness. In this sense, then, David did not really create his language, and certainly not a grammar; according to this view, a preexisting grammatical system or template directed the way he constructed his gestures, implying that his grammar did not emerge but only became manifest. Goldin-Meadow, of course, has repeated essentially this assertion in other well-known studies (e.g., Goldin-Meadow & Mylander, 1998).

This is precisely what Hopper (1987), in proposing that grammar is emergent, argues against. Such a view of language

> provides for a logically prior—perhaps eventually even biologically prior—linguistic system which is simultaneously present for all speakers and hearers, and which is a pre-requisite for the actual use of a language. It is, in other words, the scenario that when we speak we refer to an abstract, mentally represented rule system, and that we in some sense "use" already available abstract structures and schemata. (140–141)

The alternative explanation that we offer here invokes the processes of ritualization. As we have seen, once a behavior or gesture is emancipated from its external stimulus—once it becomes ritualized—as a matter of course it becomes less externally motivated and more sensitive to constraints internal to a system. We suggest that standards of well-formedness in David's gestures are emergent properties of a system undergoing ritualization, meaning that repetition, the prime mover of ritualization, would be required for the standards to appear. As the title of their article—"Once Is Not Enough"—suggests, this is precisely what the authors conclude: "These findings suggest that it is possible for an individual to introduce standards of form within a communications system, although it appears to require a period of time, perhaps years, for such standards to evolve" (Singleton, Morford, & Goldin-Meadow, 1993: 710). It scarcely needs to be added that a true nativist position, invoking a universal grammar template in the brain, would lead to the expectation of nearly instant adoption of such standards. We will consider a quite different interpretation of this sort of linguistic emergence on the part of isolated deaf signers in chapter 7 (Fusellier-Souza, 2006).

Our position is that the ontogenetic scenario we have presented here has implications for the phylogenesis of language as well. The scenario we have presented suggests that we need not believe that language or grammar are innate predispositions of the brain—structure need not be innately specified. Instead, innate predispositions of the brain to produce language—and the human brain surely differs from all other brains to some extent in this regard—are more like developmental engines (Gómez, 1997). What is selected for is not a grammatical system innately specified in each adult brain but a developmental trajectory. Bybee makes a similar point regarding the underlying cause of linguistic universals, noting that "since patterns of change cannot in themselves exist in speakers' minds, the more basic universals must be the mechanisms that create the changes that are so similar across languages" (2003, 146). The final outcome, the adult behavior, then is due to an individual with certain general cognitive abilities (and limitations) interacting with other members of his or her social group and with his or her environment. We suggest that the process of ritualization, which relies critically both on interaction with the social and physical environment and on general cognitive abilities, provides a mechanism for this developmental trajectory. In the next chapter, we explore the nitty-gritty and linguistic significance of the literal physical embodiment of language in the visual modality and how this influences the aforementioned trajectory of linguistic development.

FIVE

Conceptual Spaces and Embodied Actions

1 The Specter of Iconicity

Is language best understood as a closed, formal system designed primarily for the mental manipulation of arbitrary symbols, or is it best understood as embodied, as inextricably intertwined with the social and physical environments that provide the matrices within which it is used? Something like this question has been at the heart of much recent debate in linguistics, as was exemplified in our discussion of the Cartesian versus the cognitive-functional approaches to language.

It seems fitting in many ways that signed languages should provide the test case for the proposition that languages can be described strictly as formal symbolic systems. Beginning with Stokoe's publication of *Sign Language Structure* in 1960, it has been an uphill struggle for several generations of linguists, increasingly deaf linguists and hearing linguists with native or near-native signing ability, to convince the intellectual establishment, the general public, and the educational establishment (perhaps in that order) that the signed languages of deaf people are real languages that can be used effectively in the education of deaf children. In chapter 1, we discussed the eclipse of signed languages in the education of the deaf by strictly oralist approaches. Here we discuss how they were restored to prominence and the impact this has had on fundamental ideas about just what language is. Finally, we relate this paradigm shift to our central thesis.

The route usually taken in the quest to restore the legitimacy of signed languages has been to show that they are just like spoken languages in the terms of traditional structural/formalist linguistics—that is, that there are no important differences between speech and sign. Over the past several years, however, approaches to the linguistic study of signed languages have appeared that exploit what should have been obvious differences between languages in the visual and acoustic media. Some linguists now have confidence that they do not have to be preoccupied with rear-guard actions against reactionary educators, and that they can focus on immensely more intellectually interesting questions concerning exactly what signed languages have to tell us about the nature of language itself.

If signed languages are really languages and the human capacity for language depends on the unfolding of a genetically determined bioprogram, then we should find that the structural elements and the way they are assembled should be identical regardless of the medium, optic or acoustic, that the language user employs. On the other hand, if we believe that what makes a language a language is its fulfillment of a human need to communicate and think about certain kinds of socially important information, that is, if it is identified by its function, then we might expect that the obvious differences in medium between signed and spoken languages would be reflected in different structural arrangements. On the surface, it would seem that questions like these should be easily resolvable by empirical observation. However, in this as in many other fields of human behavior, there is a good deal of room for interpretation, and the debate has only intensified in recent years. Of course we have also been arguing that facts concerning and interpretations of the nature of signed languages have also reemerged as pivotal points in investigations of where linguistic signs and the grammatical rules that assemble them into languages come from ultimately in both phylogenetic and ontogenetic terms.

A principal fact about signed languages that has been at the core of much controversy is iconicity, or the "specter of iconicity": if true language depends on the separation of form and meaning, or *double articulation*, then to the extent that a communication system is iconic, less arbitrary, it is less a true language. Whether understood in terms of Saussure's arbitrariness of the sign or in terms of double articulation, iconicity has been a cross to bear for sign linguists since they began telling the world that signed languages are not merely mimetic gestures but true languages.

The fact that many signs of signed languages appeared to imitate in some way, by shape or movement, the things that they were intended to represent was taken as a mark of primitiveness or inferiority to speech. According to Taub,

for a long time, the doctrine of the "arbitrariness of the sign,"
attributed to de Saussure has held sway in linguistics. . . .
Symbolic forms, no longer restricted by the need to physically
resemble their referents, are what allow us to talk about
everything from amnesia to ethics. . . . According to this view,
iconic forms are limited to playacting, imitations, and the rare
onomatopoeic word, and their meanings can never be sophisticated or abstract in any way. (2001: 2)

Given this sort of bias among linguists, and, perhaps, the general public, it was natural that the linguistic study of signed language would begin
with attempts to show that the abstract and arbitrary features of phonology and syntax could be discovered and described in signed languages just
as they had been for spoken languages. Beginning with Stokoe (1960), this
is just what the linguists studying these languages attempted to do. Although the existence of iconicity was noted, it is arguable that most linguists were more interested in explaining it away than in treating it as
fundamental.

In their attempts to rid signed languages of this specter of iconicity,
linguists have taken several approaches. First, they pointed out, iconicity
appears to decrease over time: historical change in signed languages makes
them less iconic, more arbitrary (Frishberg, 1975). Second, they demonstrated that iconicity does not appear to afford much advantage for the child
who is learning a signed language (Meier, 1991). Third, they showed that
the iconicity of a sign can be submerged by the grammar—the classic demonstration being that the ASL sign SLOW, when inflected to mean VERY
SLOW, is actually signed *very fast* (Klima & Bellugi, 1979). We will consider this demonstration in detail later in this chapter. Fourth, the spec-
ter-killing linguist pointed out that knowing what a sign means does not
allow us to predict what the iconic sign might look like; conversely, seeing the sign does not necessarily allow us to predict its meaning. Although
we can see an iconic relationship in signs after we know what they mean,
it is not apparent beforehand.

Throughout the four decades of linguistic attention to signed languages,
there has been, however, an undercurrent of concern about just what iconicity
actually *does* represent in *linguistic* terms. Both Sarah Taub (2001) and
Phyllis Perrin Wilcox (2000) have recently chronicled the history of this early
interest in iconicity. For example, Wilcox (38) quotes a 1982 statement of
McDonald (1982: 12) on the significance of iconic classifiers in ASL:

The goals of a classification of ASL iconic devices are very
similar to those of standard linguistic analysis—to predict
existing forms and their distribution, and to screen out non-
occurring or non-allowed forms. In fact, we have contentions

that standard linguistic analysis *cannot* accomplish its goal with regard to these data in ASL and that recourse to a "taxonomy of iconicity" or a "visual analogue system" is absolutely necessary for the explanation and elegant description of forms in ASL.

Claims such as these continued to be fairly rare, until by the early 1990s there had arisen a chorus of discontent with the application of strict formalist linguistic principles in the study of signed languages. Taub (2001: 41) lists a number of contributors from this era, including Liddell, Van Hoek, Sherman and Phyllis Wilcox, and Brennan—all investigators who, according to Taub, began to apply the principles of the growing field of cognitive linguistics to the study of signed languages. We can add the name of Stokoe himself to this list, for his article on semantic phonology (1991) that we refer to throughout this book. Although Stokoe did not draw explicitly on ideas from cognitive linguistics, he did draw on what must be considered a precursor of this field, generative semantics, in developing his ideas on semantic phonology. We can also add to the list the French linguist Danielle Bouvet, who used both Stokoe's semantic phonology and cognitive linguistics in formulating a description of LSF signs in 1997.

Cognitive linguistics grew, beginning roughly around 1980, out of the heated debate within the field over the question whether meaning (semantics) or the formal organizing force of phonology and grammar (syntax) was more fundamental as a governing principle (see Harris, 1993). We will show here that the cognitivist framework can be applied most productively to questions concerning the description of signed language signs as well as the grammatical processes at work in ASL and other signed languages.

2 A Taxonomy of Iconicity

As we suggested, the question of the centrality of iconicity and indexicality has been a nagging one in the linguistics of signed languages, almost from the beginning of modern attempts to describe these languages in linguistic terms. Instead of avoiding the obvious iconic motivation of many signs, Bouvet (1997) uses the motivation as an aid in describing and understanding the nature of the languages that employ it. In order to make clear the full significance of this approach to describing a signed language, we must make a brief digression on the history of attempts to describe signed languages, beginning with Stokoe's initial analysis.

As we pointed out in chapter 1, the first step Stokoe took in his attempt to show that ASL was a real language was to devise a system for describing it "phonologically." It is perhaps the most basic tenet of modern structuralist/generative linguistics that languages have double articulation or duality of patterning, meaning that they are made up of a finite number of meaningless elements (phonemes) that are assembled by a set of phonological rules into meaningful units (morphemes or words), which in turn are subject to assembly into larger units by means of grammatical or syntactic rules. The phonological level is assumed to be independent of the higher levels at which meaningful sentences are constructed. It is immediately evident that the phonological level so conceived is inherently binary (thus digital)—a speech sound in any language must be meaningless, it can belong to only one phoneme class, and it cannot be intermediate in some way between two classes.

When he set about devising his descriptive system, Stokoe immediately confronted the problem that ASL is expressed in the three dimensions of visible space and thus can employ elements simultaneously, while speech is essentially linear, the sounds being expressed one at a time. Stokoe here describes how he overcame this problem (1980: 369):

> Signs cannot be performed one aspect at a time, as speakers can utter one segment of sound at a time. Signers can of course display handshapes of manual signs ad libitum, but they cannot demonstrate any significant sign action without using something to make that action somewhere. By an act of the imagination, however, it is possible to "look at" a sign as if one could see its action only or its active element only or its location only. In this way three aspects of a manual sign of sign language are distinguished, not by segmentation, it must be reemphasized, but by imagination; these were called the aspects dez (the designator, what acts), sig (signation, the action), and tab (the tabula, the place).

Problems arise almost immediately if one wishes to show identity between this system and the descriptive phonological systems of spoken languages. With respect to the issue of double articulation, for example, it cannot be maintained that these elementary aspects of signs are themselves meaningless. Dez generally refers to handshapes, and it is clear that these are often meaningful, as in the "F" handshape, indicating something grasped between the index and thumb, or the "C" handshape, indicating a cylindrical object. Moreover, with respect to the sig, the actions of many signs are clearly analogous to actual paths taken by the things referred to, and these actions are extraordinarily difficult to represent with anything resembling a binary system.

Numerous attempts to revise the system so as to get around these problems followed, but no system analogous in every way to the phonology of speech was completely satisfactory. The frustration of a developer of one of the most comprehensive attempts at a sign phonology is expressed as follows (Liddell, 2002: 75 and cited in chapter 3):

> Signers know where things are and direct signs toward them through the ability to point. The handshapes, orientation of the hand(s), the type of movement (straight, arc) are linguistically defined. The directionality of the signs is not linguistically defined. It is variable, depending completely on the actual or conceptualized location of the entity the sign is directed toward. . . . There are more than fifteen distinct proposals attempting to provide grammatical explanations for verb directionality. Only one, Liddell and Johnson (1989), attempts to provide a phonological system capable of encoding spatial loci. Even this complex system is inadequate to the task.

It was at least partly in response to what Stokoe saw as the needless complexity of the systems ASL phonologists devised that he introduced semantic phonology, wherein he suggested that his original three aspects of a sign could in fact be reduced to two, something acting and its action, and that the iconicity of the signs should be embraced, not avoided.

Acting on Stokoe's suggestions in his article on semantic phonology (1991), Bouvet (1997) shows that this can be done by analyzing the nature of the motivational linkages between iconic signs and their referents. In this case, the language in question is the one that the deaf citizens of France use as a primary language, LSF. Bouvet points out that there is no such thing as a purely iconic gestural sign, one that reproduces in every detail the object or action it is meant to denote. Instead, the symbolic relationship between an iconic sign and its referent depends on a "recognition code," and this will generally involve what the human beings inventing the sign see as the most salient feature of the thing denoted (all translations into English are by David Armstrong). Elsewhere, we discuss this process in terms of "construal." The LSF sign for "helicopter" provides an initial example. As described by Bouvet, this sign is made by placing a fluttering "3" hand above the upwardly extended index finger of a stationary "1" hand, the "3" hand clearly representing the blades of the helicopter's rotor and the "1" hand its shaft (see fig. 5.1). This sign is obviously quite similar to its ASL equivalent, a "5" hand being substituted for the "3" hand in ASL.

We described the sign for "helicopter" as "an initial example" because signs like it constitute the most basic class in Bouvet's taxonomy of LSF signs derived from their modes of production. This class is described as "descriptive signs" that "retain from the recognition code of the object being denoted, traits relative to the characteristic movement of the object and its form" (Bouvet, 1997, 24). Among the signs so classified are the follow-

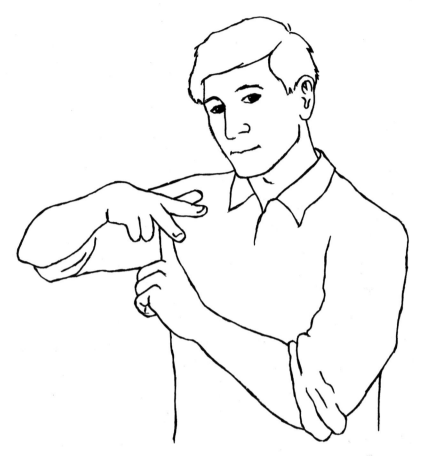

Figure 5.1. "Helicopter" in LSF. Drawing by Robert C. Johnson.

ing (many having ASL cognates): *boat, elevator, rocket, jump* (verb), *walk* (verb), *window*. Bouvet derives her taxonomy from Stokoe's semantic phonology, the insight that many iconic manual signs can be described as a "marriage of a noun and a verb"—something acting and its action. So Bouvet's taxonomy follows naturally from the mode of production of signs— it classifies them by form and movement, but not according to phonological considerations of handshape, position, and so on. Instead the classification follows the extent to which their form and movement are based on resemblance to the thing being represented, and the nature of the linkage between sign and denotatum. According to this logic, Bouvet's second and third categories of descriptive signs are those that retain either the recognition code relative to the movement made by the object or the recognition code relative to its form, but not both. In the former category are signs for things such as ladder, sweep, car, and so on that have a characteristic movement associated with them, while the latter category of signs represents objects such as bottle, chimney, roof, and so on that have a characteristic form but may not have a characteristic movement.

Within these basic categories, Bouvet creates subcategories, based, for example, on whether or not the iconic representation is done by means of a diagram or a model. Other general motivational categories follow, the next being what Bouvet calls "indicative signs," which, in turn, are divided among those that are "ostensive" (mostly naming body parts by pointing to them); "figurative" (e.g., signs for clothing where the sign is made by modeling some aspect of the clothing at the place on the body where it would be worn—as in "buttons"); or "spatial" (e.g., "down," "here"). The categories of signs discussed to this point rely on the body itself as a direct source of reference and some action of the hands that directly represents in some way the thing referred to. Bouvet moves next to processes by which more abstract entities may be represented, processes she refers to as based on "tropes," or metaphorical and other figurative processes. According to Bouvet, "tropes arise from mental associations that lead to changes in the meanings of words. They can be divided into three fundamental types: metonymy, synecdoche, and metaphor" (1997, 46). We will not go into the sometimes arcane distinctions that have been made among these categories of figurative language—suffice it to say that Wilbur (1987), P. P. Wilcox (2000), and Taub (2001) have productively applied these terms to signed languages signs and grammar, at least by analogy, and we will explore this work in much more detail later in this chapter.

Cognitive linguistics has also made productive use of these terms in descriptions of spoken languages. Bouvet presents some examples from Mark Johnson's book *The Body in the Mind* (1987). A familiar one is described as "more is up" (and less is down), so that we get expressions such as "prices are going up" ("les prix montent") and "his prestige is growing" ("son prestige grandit"). This is an example of a fundamental mental associative process that is very productive of verbal expressions, at least among speakers of French and English, and Bouvet shows that it carries over into the production of LSF signs such as "more" ("plus"), "less" ("moins"), and "too much ("trop"). Note that these are signs that directly represent the underlying metaphor as a visual image (up for more, down for less). Bouvet discusses also the metaphorical value of placing signs at various locations on the face and torso. A question that naturally arises from all of this is the following: Are there any LSF signs that can be said not to be motivated in one of the ways described here—either by direct representation or through some sort of figurative process?

Bouvet does not address this question specifically, but it is clear that she believes that signed languages are fundamentally motivated. She resolves the issue of motivation and its relation to arbitrariness within a linguistic context in the following manner:

The fact that gestural signs—whether they are concrete or abstract—are derived from processes consisting of meaningful images does not lead to their transparency by allowing the signifier to emerge directly from the signified. As with spoken languages, gestural languages must be learned, they are the products of consensus by a social group.

Thus, the phenomenon of motivation does not necessarily imply predictability, in contrast to the positions taken by structural linguistics which refers to arbitrariness when in fact phenomena are not predictable and links inversely motivation and predictability: in cognitive linguistics things are not this entrenched: "something in language or thought is motivated when it is neither arbitrary nor predictable," states G. Lakoff. (1987: 88)

In her detailed analysis of LSF, Bouvet deals only with the description of individual signs. In the next section we will show that iconicity is pervasive in the grammars of signed languages as well, with examples coming from ASL.

3 Cognitive Iconicity

Over the past decade, Wilcox (1993, 1998, 2001, 2004a, 2004b) has been developing a model of iconicity called *cognitive iconicity* based on the theory of cognitive grammar (Langacker, 1987, 1991a, 1991b, 2000). As we have seen, cognitive grammar claims that lexicon and grammar are fully describable as assemblies of symbolic structures, pairings of semantic and phonological structures. From the cognitive grammar perspective, grammar is not distinct from semantics. That is, this approach does not posit the fundamental separation between form and meaning that is the hallmark of the generative approach. Instead, the elements of grammatical description reduce to form-meaning pairings.

A critical claim of cognitive grammar is that both semantic and phonological structures reside within semantic space, which is itself a subdomain of conceptual space. Conceptual space encompasses all of our thought and knowledge, "the multifaceted field of conceptual potential within which thought and conceptualization unfold" (Langacker, 1987: 76). By adopting this view we can talk about similarities as distance between structures that reside in multidimensional conceptual space. Certain notions reside close to each other in conceptual space because they possess certain similarities. Other notions reside farther apart in conceptual space, reflecting their dissimilarity. The cognitive scientist Peter Gärdenfors (2004) proposes a similar model in which conceptual spaces representing information on the conceptual level are analyzed according to geometric principles such as closeness and betweenness; similarity of concepts, for example, is analyzed in terms of distance in conceptual space.

What is critical for cognitive iconicity is that phonological notions also reside in conceptual space. These concepts range from fairly specific, such as the way the word "dog" is pronounced by a specific speaker at a certain time with his or her distinct tone of voice, to fairly schematic, such as the way *verb* is pronounced—not a specific verb such as "throw" but the grammatical category of verb, the way *all* verbs are pronounced. Of course, for languages such as English there is no aspect of pronunciation common to all verbs or even to a set of verbs. As we will see, however, the same is not true for some signed languages such as ASL, where all verbs may have some aspect of their production in common.

The typical case for language is that semantic space and phonological space reside in vastly distant regions of conceptual space. The sound of the spoken word "dog," for example, has little in common with the meaning of the word. According to the cognitive iconicity model, this great distance in conceptual space and the resulting incommensurability of semantic and phonological space is the basis for Saussure's "l'arbitraire du signe." Alternatively, when phonological and semantic spaces reside in the same region of conceptual space, arbitrariness is reduced.

Thus cognitive iconicity is defined not as a relation between the form of a sign and what it refers to in the real world, but as a relation between two conceptual spaces. Cognitive iconicity is a distance relation between the phonological and semantic poles of symbolic structures such as words and morphemes.

Two further notions are necessary to understand how cognitive iconicity works. The first is *construal*. The mapping relation in cognitive iconicity is not between objectively defined forms and objectively determined scenes. As Langacker points out (1991b: 284), there are many ways to construe an event, and an event's objective properties are insufficient to predict its construal. This applies as well to the conception of articulatory events such as the handshapes and movements of signs. Objective properties, whether of events in the world or of articulatory events, play little role in cognitive iconicity. Iconicity is not a relation between the objective properties of a situation and the objective properties of articulators. Rather, the iconic relation is between construals of real-world scenes and construals of form. Thus, it is a selection process, similar to that invoked by Bouvet under the rubric "recognition code."

Second, we must note that metaphor can create an iconic mapping that did not exist prior to the metaphorical mapping. Because metaphor is a mapping across semantic domains, it can reposition the semantic pole of a symbolic structure to a different region of conceptual space, bringing it closer to a particular region of phonological space. For example, if in some signed language, time were conceived as a process and expressed phonologically as a handshape (an object instantiated in three-dimensional space), there would be no iconic relation: processes and objects are too distant in conceptual space to motivate cognitive iconicity. If instead time is metaphorically conceived as an object moving in space and realized phonologically as a moving handshape, the sign would be iconic. Borrowing a metaphor from cosmology, we can think of metaphor as a "worm hole" in multidimensional conceptual space. By mapping the semantics of time onto our conception of a moving object, metaphor folds conceptual space onto itself so as to bring the semantic pole of time into proximity with its phonological realization as a hand moving in signing space.

An example from ASL will help to demonstrate. As we mentioned, one common claim of traditional linguistics is that grammar in ASL submerges iconicity (Klima & Bellugi, 1979). The example that is offered to support this claim is the morphological marking of intensification on certain signs in ASL. This marking is expressed in articulation as an initial hold of the sign's movement followed by sudden, rapid release. When this grammatical marker appears on the ASL sign SLOW, the resulting sign means "very slow." Klima and Bellugi point out that because of the articulation change, the sign VERY-SLOW is made with a fast movement—faster than that used in the sign SLOW: "Thus the form of 'very slow' is incongruent with the meaning of the basic sign" (30). It is this fact that supports their claim that the grammar has submerged iconicity: "One of the most striking effects of regular morphological operations on signs is the distortion of form so that iconic aspects of the signs are overridden and submerged" (30).

A cognitive iconicity analysis leads to a different conclusion. First, note that VERY-SLOW is multimorphemic, consisting of the root lexical morpheme SLOW and a bound, grammatical morpheme marking intensification. The same bound morpheme appears on other lexical roots, such as VERY-SMART and VERY-FAST.

While it is true that the form of VERY-SLOW is incongruent with the meaning of the lexical root SLOW, the form of the intensifier morpheme is *not* incongruent with its meaning. In fact, it is highly iconic. To see this, we must note two facts about the conceptualization of intensity. Intensity is a conceptually dependent notion: intensity depends on a prior conception of what is being intensified. Something is "very *slow*" or "very *big*" but not simply "very." Second, the abstract notion of intensity is often understood metaphorically by reference to more grounded concepts such as the buildup and sudden release of internal pressure, as happens when we shake a soda can and then pop it open: the rapid movement in this case results in a face full of soda. Kövecses (2002) notes that one folk understanding of anger involves a cognitive model in which intensity of offense outweighs intensity of retribution, creating an imbalance that causes anger. As a result, a common cross-linguistic metaphorical expression of anger involves the conceptual metaphor ANGRY PERSON IS A PRESSURIZED CONTAINER.

How then is the form VERY-SLOW iconic? First, it is iconic because the articulators directly represent the metaphoric conceptualization of intensity as a sudden release of pent-up pressure: this bound morpheme is expressed as an initial hold followed by sudden release and movement. The same iconic-metaphorical expression of intensity occurs in speech. Bolinger (1986: 19) describes what he calls a "vocalized gesture" of *delayed release,* in which the initial consonant of a word is given extra length and the following vowel is cut short, as in *I'd like to wring his n-n-n-neck!* The effect is clearly one of intensification. Second, intensity as a conceptually dependent notion is also iconically represented: change in *how* the sign's movement is articulated is conceptually dependent because it relies on a prior conception of *what* movement was produced in this way.

We must also point out that this example of "submerged" iconicity is much cited in the absence of other examples. The sole reason that this example works as a demonstration of the submerging of iconicity is because of the peculiar and unique relation of the form of movement of this particular sign—a very fast motion—and the meaning of the entire construction—"very slow." This unique relation is surely the exception that proves the rule. A clear bottom line has emerged after four decades of research on signed languages: they are virtually never "counter-iconic."

What we find, then, is that a reexamination of iconicity according to the cognitive iconicity model leads to three conclusions. First, whether or not it can be shown that grammar may sometimes submerge iconicity, iconicity clearly also *emerges* on the more grammatical elements of morphologically complex forms. Second, analyzing iconicity requires that we examine our conceptualization not just of objects and events in the world but also of the articulators—hands and movements—that are the phonological pole of signed languages. Third, the iconic mapping of form and meaning in some cases is created by a metaphoric mapping.

4 Conceptualizing the Articulators

By grounding grammar in embodied conceptualization, cognitive grammar provides a link between our perception of the world as populated by objects moving through space and time and the grammatical categories and constructions used to represent these same ideas. Cognitive grammar also provides an essential element for describing cognitive iconicity—a framework for conceptualizing the articulators of signed languages. Since signed languages are produced by hands moving in space and time and perceived visually, the same theoretical constructs that are used to describe semantic structures can describe the hands as objects of conceptualization within a linguistic system.

As we discussed in section 2, Stokoe (1960) identified three major aspects of sign formation: handshape, movement, and location. Battison (1978) added a fourth, orientation (the direction in which the palm faces). Certain conceptual properties of signed language articulators are discernable:

1. The hands are autonomous objects manifest in the spatial domain.
2. Location is a dependent property, manifest in the spatial and temporal domain.
3. Orientation is a dependent property of handshapes, manifest in the spatial domain.
4. Movement is a dependent property of handshapes, manifest in the temporal domain.

Setting aside location for the moment, signs are prototypical instances of two major conceptual constructs of cognitive grammar: things (handshapes) and processes (movement). Hands are prototypical objects in interaction, either with other hands or other objects.

The location parameter spans the spatial and temporal domains. Locations have no overt articulatory manifestation; it is only by being the setting for objects that locations become manifest. The objects so located may be either actual (e.g., a handshape produced in a certain location) or virtual; when a location is virtual, it must be indicated phonologically in some way, such as a deictic gesture of the hand or eyes.

Phonological locations also may have a temporal dimension—a change in location. Change in phonological location may be used to represent a change in conceptual location; this change may either be actual or metaphorical. Change in location may be construed metaphorically as movement through space or time. It will be obvious in the following discussion that location is a rich source of grammatical iconicity, but we will not explore the topic further here (see Wilcox, 2002). The temporal dimension of location is quite a bit more complicated than discussed here. Path movement, for example, may be construed as a change in location (consider the sign GIVE) when it moves between two or more points. When the movement is circular (along a circular path), location may be construed as the setting for a movement viewed holistically rather than as a change of location (e.g., ALWAYS). Location may also be construed as a setting not only in static cases where it is the location in which a handshape occurs or point toward but also when a handshape rapidly changes due to reduplication (tremor or flutter). In the latter case, location has a dynamic aspect. Wilbur (1987: 81–84) provides a phonological analysis along these lines.

Schematicity and *specificity* are also critical aspects of cognitive iconicity. In most instances of cognitive iconicity it is necessary to describe specific construed properties of handshapes or of movements—specific handshapes and their features, specific movements with associated manners of movement, paths, and so forth—in order to discover their similarity to semantic structure. In some cases, however, such as when the semantic pole of a symbolic structure is itself highly schematic, cognitive iconicity will depend on a correspondingly schematic phonological structure. Such is the case with the iconic mapping of grammatical classes.

5 Embodied Conceptual Models

Two idealized cognitive models provide the theoretical apparatus for conceptualizing the articulators of signed languages. These are the *billiard ball model*, which describes the structure of events and provides the framework for understanding grammatical constructs such as nouns and verbs, and the *stage model*, which links our conceptual abilities to perceptual abilities. Both models are grounded in everyday experience and form the embodied basis of our conception of the world.

The billiard ball model encapsulates our conception of the world as being populated by discrete physical objects capable of moving about through space and making contact with one another (Langacker, 1991b: 13). The billiard ball model also captures the nature of *dependency relations* between objects and interactions (Langacker, 1991b). Objects can be conceptualized independently of their interactions: we can conceive of billiard balls independently of their energetic interactions on a pool table. Interactions, on the other hand, do not exist entirely independently of their participants. The conception of an interaction inherently presupposes the entities through which it is manifested. Objects are *conceptually autonomous*, and interactions *conceptually dependent* (14).

The stage model (Langacker, 1991b: 284) captures certain aspects of our conceptual abilities by relating them to perceptual experience. We can think of this as the experience of a theatergoer watching the action taking place on a stage. The observer gazes outward and focuses attention on a particular region, the stage. On stage, actors move about and handle various props. Action on stage is organized temporally into events. The stage model works in conjunction with the billiard ball model, which captures the nature of the moving participants being observed. The visual perception of these moving objects forms the basis of *role archetypes,* on which semantic roles such as agent and patient are built (fig. 5.2).

Because they reflect our experience as mobile and sentient creatures who interact with and manually manipulate physical objects (Langacker, 1991b: 285), these conceptual archetypes ground our conceptual abilities

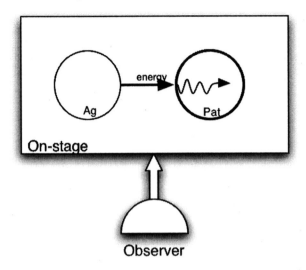

Figure 5.2. Billiard ball and stage models. "Ag" represents "Agent"; "Pat" represents "Patient."

in visual perceptual and motoric abilities. Their appearance at the heart of grammar suggests that embodied conceptual abilities, rather than abstract, modality-independent and purely linguistic abilities, account for the commonalities that we see across signed and spoken languages. It was the evolutionary development of these embodied conceptual abilities, we suggest, rather than some sudden mutation resulting in a language-specific grammar ability that led to the emergence of language. The ability to conceptualize in this way has obvious advantages for hominids whose lives were socially organized to accomplish a hunter-gatherer-forager economy.

6 Cognitive Iconicity and Signed Language Grammar

In the following sections we offer data from ASL to demonstrate the ways iconicity is pervasive in various facets of grammar: polymorphemic classifier predicates; atemporal and temporal relations; and grammatical classes.

6.1 Hands as Things, Movement as Process: Complex Polymorphemic Forms

One way handshapes represent things, and movement represents process in signed languages, is their use in so-called classifier predicates. Frishberg first introduced the term "classifier" to describe a particular type of predicate in ASL in which a handshape is used to express a verb of motion. In ASL, the verb MEET is performed by bringing the two hands together so that the knuckles meet, with the index fingers extended:

> ASL uses certain hand-shapes in particular orientations for certain semantic features of noun arguments. Thus the verb MEET has no "neutral" form: the citation form actually means "one person meets one person," or perhaps more specifically "one self-moving object with a dominant vertical dimension meets one self-moving object with a dominant vertical dimension." If trees started walking, they would MEET one another in the same way. Many of these classifiers are productive and analyzable, although not strictly transparent. (1975: 715)

As we saw in chapter 3, classifier constructions are polymorphemic forms consisting of morphemes for movement, manner of movement, semantic characteristics of the moving object, location in space, and so forth (Engberg-Pedersen, 1993). According to Newport and Meier (1985: 885), classifier predicates exhibit the following formational patterns:

> The handshape is a classifier for the semantic category (e.g. human vs. animate nonhuman vs. vehicle) or size and shape of the moving object; the movement path (one of a small number of discretely different movements, e.g. straight vs. circular vs. arc) is a morpheme representing the path of motion of the moving object; the manner of movement is a morpheme for the manner of motion along the path (e.g. bounce vs. roll vs. random); a second handshape (typically produced on the left hand) is a classifier for a secondary object, with respect to which the primary object moves; and the placement of the second handshape along the path is a morpheme for the spatial relationship of the movement path with respect to this secondary object (e.g. from vs. to vs. past).

This description might seem to suggest that classifier predicates are used only to express the motion of physical objects. In fact, these forms can be found in metaphorical and fictive motion expressions (Taub, 2001; Wilcox, 2001), thus introducing an interaction between iconicity and metaphor.

The relation of form and meaning in Newport and Meier's description is striking. Note that across all of these forms, handshapes represent objects and their features, and movements represent motions. Classifier predicates thus exhibit a systematic pattern of iconic relations in which semantic objects, the *things* of cognitive grammar, are mapped onto handshape, and *process* is mapped onto movement.

6.2 Atemporal and Temporal Relations

In addition to mapping phonological movement to process, ASL has devices for expressing atemporal relations as well. In a conversation in ASL, a deaf woman is asked to describe the changes she has seen occur over the past several decades. She responds: MUCH CHANGE, "A lot has changed." She then describes some of the things that have changed, and concludes: CHANGE-OVER-TIME, "A slow and steady change has taken place during this time." The ASL sign meaning "change" is produced in citation form with a twisting motion of the two hands (fig. 5.3).

A pattern of iconic mapping is revealed by comparing the two forms of CHANGE. The first form of CHANGE is produced by moving the hands rapidly from their initial to final configuration, which is held for a moment before the signer continues. This form of CHANGE is a stative or simple atemporal relation. (The reader should be careful not to depend on the grammatical class of the gloss. The sign is used here not as a full verb form "to change" but as a stative "has changed.") Atemporal relations lack a positive temporal profile and rely on summary as opposed to sequential scanning. The atemporal relation views the scene holistically, designating only the final state of the overall process. The iconic mapping is apparent: by virtue of the hands moving rapidly into the final, held configuration (thus decreasing the significance of movement), the phonological structure of the sign resides in the same conceptual space as its semantic structure. It means simply "something has changed."

CHANGE-OVER-TIME is produced with a slow, steady twisting movement. CHANGE-OVER-TIME is a full verb form, a relation having a positive temporal profile whose evolution through time is portrayed by sequential scanning. Whereas the stative form CHANGE designates only the final state of a process, CHANGE-OVER-TIME designates a continuous series of states distributed over time. Again, the phonological structure reveals its iconicity: the slow twisting motion brings into prominence the sequential scanning indicative of the semantic structure of a verb. Thus, the atemporal relation form CHANGE highlights only the start and end points

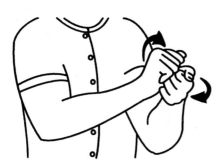

**Figure 5.3. The ASL sign
CHANGE in citation form.**

of a temporal path, while the full verb form CHANGE-OVER-TIME invites the viewer to watch all the steps along the way.

Moreover, in the form CHANGE-OVER-TIME, the twisting movement of the sign is superimposed on a slow, side-to-side movement along a sequential time-line (Engberg-Pedersen, 1993). In this way, the form iconically and metaphorically maps movement through time onto movement through space.

6.3 Aspect

Further evidence of the iconic mapping of temporal relations comes from the systematic way the ASL verb forms are grammatically marked for aspect. Comrie (1976: 3) defines aspect as "different ways of viewing the internal temporal constituency of a situation." Klima and Bellugi (1979: 292–294) describe a number of ways ASL verbs can be marked for temporal aspect. In all cases, the aspectual marking is manifest as changes to the temporal dynamics of the moving hands.

Two patterns are evident. First, aspectual marking in general is iconic: changes to the internal temporal constituency of the verb (the semantic pole) are represented by modifications to the temporal constituency of the sign's movement. Second, the iconic mapping of time extends across different aspectual forms. For example, Klima and Bellugi give the meaning of the protractive form of LOOK-AT as "to stare at (uninterruptedly)" (1979: 292–294). The semantic pole of this form represents a situation in which there is no change to the internal structure, and no well-defined end points, of the verb process. The stable situation of "looking at" persists unchanged through conceived time. This situation is described in cognitive grammar as an imperfective process in which all of the component states of a process are identical, and the verb profiles the continuation through time of a stable situation (Langacker, 1991b: 21). The semantic structure of protractive aspect in ASL is iconically represented by its phonological pole: the ASL verb form is articulated with a static form, unmoving and therefore unchanging through conceived time.

Klima and Bellugi note these patterns as well, though they make no mention of the iconicity involved (1979: 292):

> The differences in meaning indicated by inflections for different grammatical categories are mirrored by general differences in form. The most salient formal characteristic of inflections for number and distributional aspect is *spatial* patterning, with displacement along lines, arcs, and circles in vertical and horizontal planes. By contrast, inflections for temporal aspect rely heavily on *temporal* patterning, making crucial use of

dynamic qualities such as rate, tension, evenness, length, and manner in the movement of signs.

Clearly, the iconic mapping of space and time is pervasive in the grammar of ASL (see Wilcox, 2002, for further discussion).

6.4 Grammatical Classes

It would seem at first that grammatical classes such as noun and verb could not be iconically represented. There are two reasons for this. First, if we accept the traditional view of iconicity as a relation between language and the real world, we find no iconic mapping, because grammatical classes do not exist in the real world: they are purely relational phenomena within the world of language. Second, within the traditional view of language, grammatical classes cannot be defined in notional terms, and so they have no semantic pole. Even functional linguists dismiss the possibility that grammatical categories such as nouns and verbs could be accounted for solely by means of semantics (Hopper & Thompson, 1984).

It is not surprising then that signed language linguists make statements such as the following (Valli & Lucas, 1995: 7): "It is probably true that the form of the sign SIT is an iconic representation of human legs sitting. . . . [However,] focusing on its iconicity will not provide much insight into the interesting relationship between SIT and the noun CHAIR, and other noun-verb pairs."

What Valli and Lucas are claiming is that, while the shape of the hands in SIT and CHAIR may iconically represent human legs and the seat of a chair (by the first two fingers dangling over the extended fingers of the other hand), the relation between morphologically related nouns and verbs such as CHAIR and SIT is not iconically represented.

A key claim of cognitive grammar is that nouns and verbs lend themselves to schematic semantic characterization. A noun profiles a region in some domain, given the technical term *thing*. Verbs are a series of stative relations distributed continuously through conceived time, the component states viewed serially rather than holistically (Langacker, 1991a: 20–21). This relation is called a *process*. Cognitive grammar thus claims that the noun class profiles a *thing* and the verb class profiles a *process* (fig. 5.4).

As symbolic structures, noun and verb classes also have phonological poles. In most cases the phonological poles of nouns and verbs are so schematic, consisting only of some phonological specification, that they may be left unspecified, as indicated in figure 5.4 by an ellipsis at the phonological pole. If there were a regular phonological distinction marking nouns and verbs, the phonological pole would reflect this.

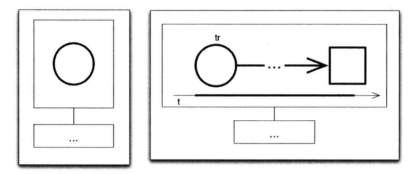

Figure 5.4. Noun schema (a) and verb schema (b).

This is the case for ASL and many other signed languages, in which a systematic phonological pattern marks certain nouns and verbs (Supalla & Newport, 1978). In ASL, for example, the noun BOOK is phonologically related to the verb OPEN-BOOK: BOOK is made with reduplicated, short movements, while OPEN-BOOK uses one long movement (fig. 5.5).

Klima and Bellugi (1979: 295–296) note that while both continuous and hold manner occur in the verb signs (a continuous sweep as opposed to a noticeable stop at the end of the movement), the noun forms have reduplicated movement and a restrained manner. As a result, the nouns are typically made with smaller movements than their related verbs.

Because these noun-verb pairs have schematic phonological specifications, they exhibit cognitive iconicity in two ways. First, these forms are often iconic for some aspect of their lexical meaning: SIT and CHAIR do iconically represent legs dangling off of the flat seat of a chair. These forms

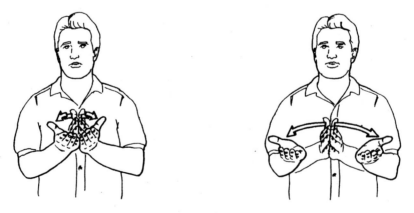

Figure 5.5. Noun-verb pairs in ASL: (a) the ASL noun BOOK; (b) the ASL verb OPEN-BOOK.

also iconically represent their grammatical class. Because of their restrained manner and reduplicated movement, noun forms are articulated in a region of conceptual space occupied by *things*. Verb forms, because of their salient movement through space, reside in the region of conceptual space occupied by *processes*.

Finally, note that this is a case where cognitive iconicity relies not on specificity at the semantic and phonological poles but on schematicity. The reason these noun-verb forms are iconic is precisely because they share highly schematic phonological characteristics with their respective schematic semantic pole—that is, what they actually represent in the real world.

We will next consider the role of iconicity and metaphorical processes in the description of sign language grammars.

7 Signing Metaphorically

Two recent books, by P. P. Wilcox (2000) and Taub (2001), address the issue of iconicity and metaphor in the grammar of ASL. The key is the cognitivist claim that a complex network of metaphorical mapping underlies the structures of our linguistic acts. Use of the term "metaphor" in cognitive linguistics is, of course, somewhat more generic than its use in literary theory and criticism, so that "metaphoric" in cognitive linguistic usage might equate in some ways with "imagistic" in ordinary usage. Wilcox and Taub each consider a variety of metaphorical pathways underlying ASL imagery, including several that have secondary iconic outcomes as described earlier: *more is up, good is up, powerful is up*. The vertical scale is, obviously, easily represented by direct action in signing. The underlying metaphors may be based on such universal experiences as piling things up as quantities increase, the fact of being vertical indicating health and strength, and dominance being reinforced by physical size. Not only are these human universals but they are certainly universal to the higher primates and, perhaps, to some extent, the vertebrate subphylum (e.g. Givens, 1986). In the case of an otherwise fairly opaque sign such as PRESIDENT in ASL, the *powerful is up* metaphor is represented in the formation of the sign in front of the forehead.

Both books also present sophisticated and well-developed schemes for analyzing signs that involve multiple metaphorical sources, for example the sign glossed as THINK-PENETRATE. In this construction, the extended index finger ("G" classifier or "1" hand) moves outward from the forehead and, upon encountering the palmar side of the other ("B") hand with its fingers extended, penetrates between the index and second fingers of it, as if penetrating a solid object. The usual translation is that this represents the successful communication of an idea to someone who is particularly resistant to receiving it. According to Taub, this sign involves metaphorical mapping from at least two source domains: "ideas can be conceived of as objects," and "communicating is sending." Taub's full analysis is presented in table 5.1 (fig. 6.6 in Taub, 2001: 103).

According to Wilcox's analysis of the same sign, THINK-PENETRATE depends on the underlying metaphors *IDEAS IN EXISTENCE ARE STRAIGHT* and *THE MIND IS A CONTAINER*. Many other examples are given to reinforce the notion that these are fundamental organizing metaphors in ASL. Some of the flavor of her formal analysis can be gathered from figure 5.6 (2000: 129).

Both authors present numerous examples such as these to support the premise that a signed language such as ASL cannot be adequately described without recourse to analysis of these underlying metaphorical structures. At the same time, both forcefully maintain that the construction of these ultimately motivated forms is highly constrained with respect to the articulators that can be employed and the mapping structures that can be followed. In other words, the output is highly conventionalized, as it would have to be in order to be comprehensible to someone receiving it.

Taub suggests explicitly that it is now time to explore what makes signed languages different from spoken languages and what may be learned from the differences (2001: 223). Taub is primarily interested in grammar, and from the following perspective—what are the rules for selection of particular iconic forms from the range of options that presents itself in any given situation? She derives rules governing this sort of choice, especially with respect to the paths of verbs that have been called "agreement verbs" in ASL.

Table 5.1. Iconic mapping of THINK-PENETRATE.

	Iconic Mapping	Metaphorical Mapping
Articulators	Source	Target
1→	An object	An idea
Forehead	Head	Mind; locus of thought
1→ touches forehead	Object located in head	Idea understood by originator
1→ moves toward locus of addressee	Sending an object to someone	Communicating idea to someone
Nondominant B	Barrier to object	Difficult in communication
1→ inserted between fingers of B	Penetration of barrier	Success in communication despite difficulty
Signer's locus	Sender	Originator of idea
Addressee's locus	Receiver	Person intended to learn idea

Source: Reprinted, by permission of the publisher, from S. Taub, *Language from the Body* (Cambridge: Cambridge University Press, 2001).

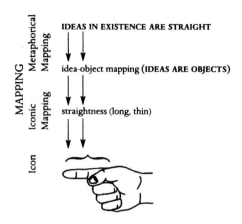

MAPPING

Metaphorical Mapping

Iconic Mapping

Icon

IDEAS IN EXISTENCE ARE STRAIGHT

idea-object mapping (IDEAS ARE OBJECTS)

straightness (long, thin)

Figure 5.6. Iconic mapping of THINK-PENETRATE. From Phyllis P. Wilcox, *Metaphor in American Sign Language* (Washington, DC: Gallaudet University Press, 2000), page 129. Reprinted with the permission of the publisher.

Unlike most previous analysts, however, Taub argues that the paths taken by ASL agreement verbs are ultimately motivated by semantic considerations and not by the rules of formal grammar, for example, movement from subject to object. In this regard, in fact, agreement verbs would seem to be fairly obviously iconically motivated. For example, the movement of the ASL verb GIVE is from the giver to the receiver, representing in a straightforwardly iconic manner the transfer of an object from one owner to another. Taub seeks to provide a framework for dealing with a class of agreement verbs in which the underlying motivation is more complex.

Taub pays particular attention to a class of agreement verbs that have been referred to as "backward." These are verbs in which movement is toward the subject—verbs such as STEAL, TAKE, and BORROW—and their action is obviously not explained by an arbitrary grammatical rule that specifies movement from subjects toward objects. Taub shows conclusively that only a semantic analysis involving iconic and metaphorical pathways provides a satisfactory explanation for the behavior of these and other verbs that involve multiple possible pathways. It is beyond the scope of this chapter to explicate fully Taub's analysis, but her analysis shows that, in general, ASL has a hierarchical structure for the selection of possible pathways. In the case of agreement verbs, the movement of an actual or metaphorical object from its source to its goal will generally determine the course of actual movement of the verb. In cases where there might be a potential conflict between possible paths, Taub identifies a hierarchical set of rules that will determine which path is chosen.

The following example illustrates the problem. There are two signs (or sentences) in ASL with very similar meanings having to do with the gathering of visual information, and glossed as I-LOOK-(AT)-HIM/HER/IT and I-PERCEIVE-BY-EYES-HIM/HER/IT. They differ with respect to the direction of action of the signs—in the former, the path is from the subject toward the object being viewed, and in the latter the action is toward the subject. The difference in meaning is what might be expected, given the iconic and metaphorical underpinnings of the two utterances. As Taub puts it, the "verbs profile slightly different parts of the [semantic] frame." In LOOK, the energy is directed outward, and in PERCEIVE-BY-EYES what is profiled is what the viewer "gets from" the picture—metaphorically, something is taken into the eyes. The direction of motion of the verbs can, thus, only be predicted from the meanings of the signs, not by an abstract grammatical rule. Taub is explicit that her ultimate goal is not to provide a set of "grammatical" rules, per se. Instead, she believes "that a good grammar of a language should not include rules; elements of the grammar should either be actual forms of the language or 'schemas' that generalize over forms of the language." The hierarchical rules referred to here can be regarded, "however, as a sort of shorthand for a full cognitive model that has not yet been worked out" (2001: 193).

Phyllis Wilcox asks this question (2000: 5): "What is a metaphor? What defines metaphoric mapping and how is it constrained? Why is there so much variation among researchers regarding the identification of metaphorical referents? Are similar referential counterparts found in ASL?" She then describes a process she refers to as removing the "shroud of iconicity" to reveal metaphorical signing. Her point is that metaphorical mapping of the kind discussed earlier has often been confused with direct iconic representation in signed languages. This is, perhaps, not surprising, as Peirce, in his original taxonomy of signs, classified metaphor as iconic. We can see how this would happen with respect to such powerful and pervasive metaphorical mappings as those that derive from the vertical scale. The idea that up is positive is so pervasive that it seems "natural," and thus iconic, that it should be reflected in signing. But there is nothing about an abstract quality such as goodness or power that can be directly represented iconically—believing that there is an example of what philosophers have called the "naturalistic fallacy"—the belief that qualities inhere in objects. Instead, positive values have come to be *associated* with the direction "up" through a sociocultural process, possibly beginning with the notion that it is "good" for a person to be able to assume a vertical position (being able to stand up reflects at least minimally good health). Similarly, there is a basic perception that a large human being or other animal is powerful, so height comes to be associated with power and dominance.

With respect to the debate over what makes a signed language a language, whether it has to meet some formal standard involving phonology, morphology, or syntax, Taub and Wilcox prove, paradoxically, that it is the application of the cognitive linguistic framework to the metaphors underlying both signed and spoken languages that reveals the fundamental unity. The unity is in the cognitive engines that drive these languages, not in the structures of their expressions at the surface in terms of gestural behavior. The unity is thus not at the phonological, morphological, or syntactic levels. What Stokoe was revealing when he showed that sign language signs can be decomposed as speech signs can was not something linguistic. Rather he was tapping into the more general tendency for all human social behavior to be conventionalized and thus structured by the winnowing-out of some possible elements and the inclusion of only a subset of others. In the following chapter, we will discuss how these iconic and metaphorical processes lead to the emergence of specific grammatical structures from gestural precursors. Language grows out of the human body interacting with its physical and social environments—metaphorical structures are the pathways from gesture to meaning.

In the next chapter, we complete the loop by showing how the study of language and gesture can be reunited in a single, powerful, evolutionary framework.

The Gesture-Language Interface

1 Reestablishing the Language/Gesture Interface

At the infamous conference held in Milan in 1880 mentioned in chapter 1, educators of the deaf from Europe and
North America met to denounce the use of signed languages in the education of deaf children. The result of this
conference was the virtual extinction of these languages as
vehicles for instruction in classrooms for deaf students for
a century. The languages lived on, but the education of
deaf children was stifled. At the Milan conference, Giulio
Tarra attempted to malign sign language by equating it with
gesture:

> Gesture is not the true language of man which
> suits the dignity of his nature. Gesture, instead of
> addressing the mind, addresses the imagination
> and the senses. Moreover, it is not and never will
> be the language of society. . . . Thus, for us it is an
> absolute necessity to prohibit that language and to
> replace it with living speech, the only instrument
> of human thought. . . . Oral speech is the sole
> power that can rekindle the light God breathed
> into man when, giving him a soul in a corporeal
> body, he gave him also a means of understanding,
> of conceiving, and of expressing himself. . . .

While, on the one hand, mimic signs are not sufficient to express the fullness of thought, on the other they enhance and glorify fantasy and all the faculties of the sense of imagination. . . . The fantastic language of signs exalts the senses and foments the passions, whereas speech elevates the mind much more naturally, with calm and truth and avoids the danger of exaggerating the sentiment expressed and provoking harmful mental impressions. (Lane, 1984: 391, 393–394)

Tarra was not alone in attempting to link gesture with sign and hence the baser aspects of human nature. He was joined by other oralist educators who believed that sign language was nothing more than gesture, and that neither was capable of serving the linguistic functions necessary to separate man from the animals. Consider this report of the remarks of Marius Magnat, the director of an oral school in Geneva at the time (Lane, 1984: 387–388):

The advantages of articulation training [i.e., speech] . . . are that it restores the deaf to society, allows moral and intellectual development, and proves useful in employment. Moreover, it permits communication with the illiterate, facilitates the acquisition of and use of ideas, is better for the lungs, has more precision than signs, makes the pupil the equal of his hearing counterpart, allows spontaneous, rapid, sure, and complete expression of thought, and humanizes the user. Manually taught children are defiant and corruptible. This arises from the disadvantages of sign language. It is doubtful that sign can engender thought. It is concrete. It is not truly connected with feeling and thought. . . . It lacks precision. . . . Signs cannot convey number, gender, person, time, nouns, verbs, adverbs, adjectives. . . . It does not allow [the teacher] to raise the deaf-mute above his sensations. . . . Since signs strike the senses materially they cannot elicit reasoning, reflection, generalization, and above all abstraction as powerfully as can speech.

By drawing the lines between sign, gesture, and the body on the one hand and speech, language, and the mind—the uniquely human—on the other, the oralists sought to banish sign language from the classroom. Unfortunately for linguists, they also contributed to a quarantine on the scientific study of the gesture-language interface that lasted for a century. In table 6.1 we list the traditional elements of this separation, elements that are traceable to at least Descartes, as we have seen throughout this book. To this, we can now add digital to the mind list and analog to the body list.

Table 6.1. Mind/body dualism in relation to language and gesture.

Mind	Body
Language	Gesture
Speech	Sign
Acquisition of ideas	Concrete
Expression of thought; instrument of thought	Cannot engender thought
Restored to society: calm, prudence, truth human-like)	Defiant, corruptible, undignified animal-like)
Precision (grammar)	Lacks grammar (number, gender, nouns, verbs, etc.); mimic
Elicits and permits reasoning, reflection, abstraction, generalization, conceptualization; rationality	Associated with the senses (sensual), material, glorifies imagination and fantasy, foments passions, encourages harmful mental impressions
The soul; the spirit	The corporeal body; the flesh; the material world

Although this quarantine has recently begun to break down and lin-guists have once again begun to examine the role of gesture in signed lan-guages, for the most part these studies still regard the two as categorically distinct though intertwined—that is, that signed languages involve blends of gestural and linguistic elements (Emmorey & Riley, 1995; Liddell, 1998; Liddell & Metzger, 1998). What we hope we have accomplished in this book is to show that the categorical distinction between language and gesture is not necessary.

In previous chapters, we have considered processes of lexicalization and grammaticization—the processes by which signals become gestures, which in turn become signs and words, which finally become complex, grammatically organized utterances. At no point in this process do we detect a categorical break between where gestures disappear and linguistic units take their place. Instead we see a never-ending evolutionary pro-cess according to which symbolic gestures are introduced into linguistic systems, are elaborated, and decay, according to processes, including ritualization, that are similar across species, but that are uniquely elabo-rated among human beings.

2 The Gesture-Sign Language Interface

A new line of research explores the process by which gesture becomes incorporated into *signed languages* (S. Wilcox, 2000, 2001; Wilcox et al.,

2000). These studies demonstrate a variety of ways gesture appears with and becomes a part of signed languages. The evidence from this research suggests that nonlinguistic gestures first become incorporated as lexical signs in a particular signed language.

For example, the gesture "come here" is commonly used among hearing people; it was identified as long ago as 1832 by de Jorio as functioning to call or summon someone: "Fingers extended and then brought towards the palm several times." This gesture has become incorporated into signed languages, for example, in Catalan Sign Language with the meaning "emergency," and in old ASL with the meaning "necessity" (Higgins, 1923). Pragmatic inferencing, which has been shown to play a critical role in semantic change in spoken languages (Traugott, 1989), may be invoked to explain the process by which this gesture has lexicalized: one reason a person would beckon another to come is because of an urgent need.

Research on spoken languages demonstrates that lexical material may further evolve into grammatical elements of a language by the process of grammaticization (Bybee et al., 1994). One example of this is the English lexical verb "go," which has in addition to its lexical sense of movement in space a grammatical sense that is used to mark tense, typically pronounced "gonna": "I'm gonna fly to New York next week."

It now appears that gestures, in addition to lexicalizing, may undergo further development in signed languages and acquire grammatical function. The process by which this happens is called grammaticization. Numerous scholars have described grammaticization as synonymous with the evolutionary process of ritualization: "In the course of evolution, both locomotory movements and acts . . . have been selected and modified to produce signals" (Blest, 1963: 102). Haiman notes that this process "amounts to *the creation of (a) language out of other kinds of behavior"* (1998b: 141). Ritualization thus is implicated in the phylogenetic evolution of language from nonlinguistic behaviors, among which visible-manual gestures played a key role. Ritualization is also implicated in the origins of sign languages, with lexicalization and grammaticization of gesture playing a significant role in their ongoing development. What appears unique about signed languages, when they are compared to spoken languages, is the transparency of this process to observers. In the following section we describe two routes by which gesture develops into grammatical forms in signed languages.

3 Two Routes from Gesture to Language

Attitudes toward signed languages such as those Giulio Tarra expressed not only suppressed the exploration of iconicity, they had an even more oppressive effect on the linguistic study of the relation between gesture and signed languages. The prevailing view among sign linguists is that gesture and signed language are categorically distinct, and any mention of a possible relation between the two is regarded as a challenge to the linguistic status of signed languages.

We must admit, however, that linguistic material comes from somewhere. To posit a link between gesture and signed languages, and to propose a route by which gesture becomes language, does not deny that each is unique. It merely recognizes the remarkable family resemblances between signs and gestures, hinting at a common ancestor (Armstrong et al., 1995).

Gesture follows at least two routes of incorporation into signed languages. The first route begins with a gesture that is not a conventional unit in the linguistic system. This gesture becomes incorporated into a signed language as a lexical item. Over time, these lexical elements acquire grammatical function. An example comes from the development of futures. Using a corpus of historical and modern conversational data, Shaffer and Janzen (2002) demonstrate that the grammatical morpheme marking future in ASL (fig. 6.1) developed from a lexical morpheme "go" (fig. 6.2).

The source of the "depart" morpheme appears to be a gesture described as early as de Jorio (2000 [1832]); it is produced with the palm of the hand open and held edgewise, moved upward several times. This gesture is still in use among hearing people in the Mediterranean region to signal departure-demand and departure-description (Morris et al., 1979), as shown

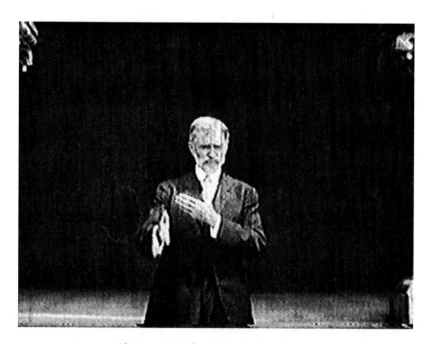

Figure 6.1. The ASL sign FUTURE.

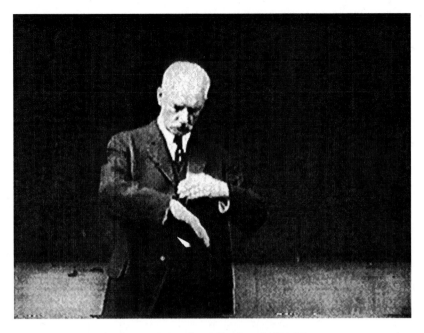

Figure 6.2. The ASL sign DEPART.

in figure 6.3 (note that figure 6.3 is not a sign language sign, it is a gesture made by a hearing person).

This gesture also appears in nineteenth-century LSF as the lexical morpheme PARTIR, "depart" (fig. 6.4).

The second route proceeds along a different path. The source is not a free-standing gesture capable of being incorporated as a lexical item into a signed language. Rather, the source gesture may be one of several types, including:

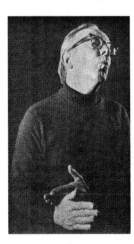

Figure 6.3. Departure-demand/description gesture. From L. Wylie and R. Stafford, *Beaux Gestes: A Guide to French Body Talk* (Cambridge: Undergraduate Press, 1977).

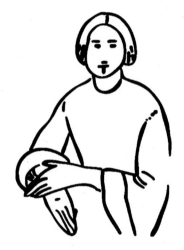

Figure 6.4. 1855 LSF lexical sign
PARTIR, "depart." From J. Brouland,
*Langage Mimique: Spécimen d'un
dictionaire des signes* (1855),
Gallaudet Archives, Gallaudet
University, Washington, DC.

1. A particular manner of movement such as that seen in the intensifier morpheme and verb aspect
2. A facial gesture such as the question markers and adverbials discussed earlier or the topic/conditional marker (Janzen et al., 2000)
3. Various mouth and eye gestures (Cagle, 2001)

As just described, these are clearly linguistic features. Support for the claim that they derive from gestural sources comes from their similarity to intonation and other verbal gestures (Bolinger, 1983, 1986); the identification of topic and conditional markers with nonlinguistic gestures marking surprise (Janzen & Shaffer, 2002); and the existence of gestures that occur in aspect-marked speech contexts (Duncan, 2002; Parrill, 2000, 2001) that are strikingly similar in form to those seen in ASL verb aspect.

These gestural types differ in the degree of schematicity of their form and meaning. Those along the first route have fairly specific phonological form, specific handshapes for example. Those along the second route are generally more schematic, both in form and meaning. Manner of movement, for example, is quite schematic in its phonological form, the particular manifestation depending on exactly which movement is being modified. The distinction parallels that between lexical and grammatical morphology. Langacker (1991b: 3) notes that the symbolic units generally analyzed as lexical items tend to be morphologically simple and quite specific in their semantic and their phonological content. The units thought of as grammatical are more schematic semantically and often phonologically; grammatical morphemes typically have specific phonological shapes but schematic meanings.

This description suggests an explanation of these two routes of development from gesture to language. In the first route, gestural elements that are fairly specific in their semantic and their phonological content become incorporated into signed languages as lexical items; these grammaticize into units that are more schematic phonologically and semantically in ways much the same as that found for spoken languages (Janzen & Shaffer, 2002; Wilcox, 2002). In the second route, gestural elements that have schematic semantic content, though fairly specific phonological content, directly take on grammatical function as they become a part of the linguistic system.

This description is entirely compatible with and predictable from the claims made in chapter 5 concerning cognitive iconicity. Visual articulators such as hands and faces come with inherent conceptual significance. The conceptual import of these articulators is not just present when they are elements in the linguistic system, but extends outside of the linguistic system to gestures. This suggests that nonlinguistic gestures may serve as sources for morphemes in signed languages, and that the specific properties of these gestures will determine their developmental path as they enter the linguistic system.

Further, we should not expect to find a categorical distinction between meaningful gestures such as those described by Calbris (1985, 1990), McNeil (1992), and Duncan (2002) and incipient morphemes of a signed language. Although gestures and signs differ, they do so along dimensions common to both and in a continuous rather than categorical way. Dimensions along which symbolic structures for language vary are likely sufficient to describe the graded development of gesture to language: symbolic complexity, specificity/schematicity, psychological entrenchment, and conventionalization.

We have already seen that specificity/schematicity is a primary factor determining the route taken as gesture is incorporated into signed languages. Symbolic complexity, the degree to which symbolic structures are decomposable into smaller symbolic elements, also may be a significant factor. McNeill (1992: 21) notes that gestures lack internal complexity: "Two gestures produced together don't combine to form a larger, more complex gesture. There is no hierarchical structure of gestures made out of other gestures." We should also note, however, that when visible gestures occur in cospeech contexts they are component elements in composite (albeit cross-modal) symbolic structures.

The primary factors distinguishing the symbolic structures of gesture and those of signed languages are psychological entrenchment and conventionality. Notably, frequency of use is a major force driving both of these factors, as it is in grammaticization.

Once a form enters the linguistic system, it can undergo grammaticization and lose its semanticity; this process can eventually erode all meaning until all that is left is meaningless form. Hopper (1994) describes this process as *phonogenesis*. Examples from ASL include the loss of semanticity when the LSF number handshapes became incorporated into certain ASL signs. In LSF, a closed handshape with extended thumb means "one" and thumb plus index finger means "two." The "one" handshape appears in the ASL signs TOMORROW, YESTERDAY, and ACCOMPANY/WITH, where it has lost its morphemic value and now exists only as a phoneme. Evidence that these ASL signs once contained the morpheme "one" comes from two sources. First, the contemporary LSF signs HIER, DEMAIN, and AVEC are cognates of the ASL signs and include the morpheme (Cuxac, 2000). Second, corresponding forms are attested in early to middle nineteenth-century LSF.

The "two" handshape appears in TWENTY, TWENTY-ONE, and THEN in ASL but does not retain the meaning of "two"; in all ASL forms except these, "two" is indicated by a V-handshape. Finally, we find evidence for person marking in old LSF "I am mistaken/you are mistaken," where the first-person/second-person distinction is indicated by location: first-person "I am mistaken" is signed near the chin, and second-person "You are mistaken" is signed at a neutral location in front of the signer (fig. 6.5). Location was morphemic in old LSF, as it is in many contemporary ASL signs marked for agreement. Only the first-person monomorphemic form remains in ASL, meaning "wrong"; the chin location is a demorphologized phoneme.

Morphemes arise and disappear in signed languages, just as they do in spoken languages. What is striking about the process for signed languages

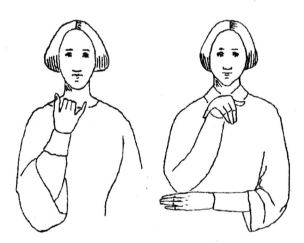

Figure 6.5. Location as morpheme in LSF: (a) "I am mistaken"; (b) "You are mistaken." From J. Brouland, *Langage Mimique: Spécimen d'un dictionaire des signes* (1855), Gallaudet Archives, Gallaudet Archives, Gallaudet University, Washington, DC.

is the source of grammatical morphemes. Meillet (1948: 131) claimed that lexical items are the only known source of grammatical morphemes. As we have seen, grammatical morphemes in signed languages arise directly from gestural sources. When gestures are the source, the articulators already possess a conceptual significance that, along with their nascent semantic structure, partially determines their semantic value when they become part of the linguistic system.

Further, even though old morphemes become meaningless phonemes through phonogenesis, they retain their inherent conceptual properties and can be recruited as meaningful again. Frozen classifiers can thaw, and poets can make creative, symbolic use of the inherent conceptual significance of hands and their movements. Just as the categorical distinction between gesture and language cannot be maintained, so the distinction between phonology and morphology is a matter of degree. Morphemes arise in a gradual fashion, and for signed languages not just from other morphemes. As Haiman (1998b: 156–157) notes:

> With insignificant exceptions like "ouch" and "boo hoo," we cannot observe how words developed out of nonwords; however far back we go, it seems that all of our etymologies of words trace to nothing but other older words. But we may be able to observe the genesis of codification in the stereotyping of intonation, which, as it has often been observed, lies at the border between paralinguistic and linguistic behavior. Although there is much stereotyping (codification) in this realm, it is inherently less digitally coded than morpho-syntax, more inherently analogic and iconic . . . and more subject to personal variation.

When we include data from signed languages we discover that gestures are a nonword source of lexical and grammatical morphemes.

In discussing the second route by which gesture becomes incorporated into signed languages, we suggested that verb aspect is linked with gesture and intonation. We are not claiming that verb aspect derives directly from the type of gesture described by Duncan and Parrill. We do claim, however, that manner of movement, which is how aspect is indicated in cospeech gestures as well as in ASL, varies along a continuum from paralinguistic to morphemic. Thus, the second route by which gesture becomes incorporated into signed languages is equivalent to the genesis of codification.

Finally, just as "creeping double articulation" (Haiman, 1998b: 149) from increasing codification occurs in spoken languages, so, too, is duality of patterning an emergent and variable property of signed languages. Partly this is due to the same factors that lead to the emergence of double articulation in spoken languages: "as signs become emancipated from, and autonomous relative to, their extralinguistic real-world referents, they may be free to become more sensitive to their linguistic context, that is, the other signs with which they co-occur" (149). For signed languages, however, this Saussurean systematicity is never devoid of the ever-present conceptual significance of visible articulators. No matter how much a sign increases its *valeur,* its relationship to other signs in the linguistic system, it can never totally sever its *signifiance,* its relationship to something in the world. Pressures internal to the linguistic system can never submerge the forces that relate signs outside of the system or to the demands of human cognition and communication.

4 Arbitrariness and Iconicity Revisited

Arbitrariness and iconicity often are regarded as mutually exclusive properties of linguistic systems. The view of cognitive iconicity proposed here does not require such an opposition; on the contrary, it permits and even predicts that arbitrariness and iconicity can be simultaneously present.

The view that arbitrariness and iconicity are mutually exclusive derives from the assumption that iconicity requires full predictability: if a form is iconic, some would claim, then we should be able to predict its form from its meaning, and vice versa. What this assumption does not take into consideration is the role of construal. Cognitive iconicity recognizes that construal operates on both poles of symbolic structures. Because of this double construal operation, a high degree of arbitrariness is always present, even when the symbolic structure is clearly iconic. As Janzen notes, "in a signed language, mapping the features of a highly subjective construal of an event onto spatial discourse features introduces a potential increase in arbitrariness in that certain aspects of the event may be profiled at the expense of others—it is the *choice* of what to profile that is arbitrary" (2004: 168).

Pietrandrea (2002) documented this fact in the Italian Sign Language (LIS) lexicon. In a study of 1,944 signs, she found that 50 percent of handshape occurrences and 67 percent of body location occurrences had an iconic motivation. Alongside this pervasive iconicity, however, exists a deep arbitrariness in the LIS lexicon, because iconic signs exhibit arbitrary selection of different aspects of articulators and referents to convey different meanings. As we pointed out in detail in the previous chapter, Bouvet makes the same claim for LSF.

A second factor that permits iconicity and arbitrariness to coexist is the inherent conceptual significance of signed language articulators. Even though symbolic structures necessarily increase in arbitrariness as they become part of the linguistic system, they nevertheless retain their inherent conceptual significance. The balance between system-internal signification and inherent conceptual significance may often tip in favor of the linguistic system, but a variety of factors can act to unleash the conceptual potential of a sign's form.

Iconicity and arbitrariness also wax and wane in another way. The erosion of iconicity in the lexicon is offset by the emergence of iconicity in the grammar, as seen in the ASL intensifier morpheme. Moreover, when gestures serve as the source of lexical and grammatical morphology, this reintroduces new iconicity into the system.

Iconicity is commonly identified as a motivation of linguistic form. Cognitive iconicity suggests an alternative view: iconicity is symptomatic of something more fundamental that unites both form and meaning. Haiman says:

> Since the transformational revolution, it has been claimed that the structure of language reflects the structure of THOUGHT, and that its study provides a "window on the mind". In arguing, as I have done, for the iconicity of grammar in general, I contend that the structure of thought in its turn reflects the structure of REALITY to an extent greater than it is now fashionable to recognize. (1980: 537)

While we may question whether iconic mappings are truly reflections of reality—iconic mappings are always between construals of form and construals of reality—iconicity does reveal the structure of conception. Iconicity is symptomatic of the underlying unity of phonological and semantic space as domains within our conceptual space. The congruence of phonological and semantic structures in iconicity emanates from a common conceptual system that underlies and gives structure to both linguistic form and meaning.

Signed languages, by using articulators that visibly manifest the same grounded archetypes that underlie our conceptual abilities—objects moving in space within our field of vision—differ from spoken languages in that they have an enhanced potential for realizing these iconic mappings. This is a fact fully compatible with a cognitive view of language, but it is certainly not a new insight. Charles Hockett (1978: 274) regarded this difference between signed and spoken languages to be one of *syntactic dimensionality,* "that is, the geometry of the field in which the constituents of a message are displayed, different arrangements often yielding different meanings." Hockett's distinction between "signages" and "languages" in the following passage is unnecessary, and his mention of pantomiming unwittingly evokes the ghosts of the aforementioned Milan conference of educators of the deaf; but his point could never be more relevant as we apply the findings of cognitive linguistics to the study of signed languages (274–275):

The difference in dimensionality means that signages can be iconic to an extent to which languages cannot. . . . Now, while arbitrariness has its points, it also has its drawbacks, so that it is perhaps more revealing to put it the other way around, as a limitation of spoken languages. Indeed, the dimensionality of signing is that of life itself, and it would be stupid not to resort to picturing, pantomiming, or pointing whenever convenient. . . . But when a representation of some four-dimensional hunk of life has to be compressed into the single dimension of speech, most iconicity is necessarily squeezed out. In one-dimensional projection, an elephant is indistinguishable from a woodshed. Speech perforce is largely arbitrary; if we speakers take pride in that, it is because in 50,000 years or so of talking we have learned to make a virtue of necessity.

In considerably less time, linguists have elevated features derived from the study of one type of language, spoken language, to the status of linguistic universals. In doing so, they have committed a cardinal scientific error: generalizing from a biased data sample. Upon reviewing the evidence from signed languages, Hockett discarded the design feature that all language is transmitted in the vocal-auditory channel. The data presented here suggest that it is time for linguists to reexamine the role of vision, iconicity, and gesture in the grammars of signed languages and the implications of this for the evolution of language in general.

We conclude our argument by considering historical evidence concerning the visual basis for the emergence and evolution of languages. It is often maintained that theories of the evolution of language are purely speculative "just-so" stories. In our concluding chapter, we show that this assumption is untrue. Evidence concerning stages in the emergence of two forms of visually based language—writing and the signed languages of the deaf—confirms major aspects of the gestural origin theory that we have presented in this book. Significantly, we show that this evidence supports Stokoe's original insights into the theoretical construct he called "semantic phonology."

SEVEN

Invention of
Visual Languages

Our argument to this point has been largely speculative, although we have presented direct evidence concerning the processes of grammaticalization in signed languages that supports the notion that these languages are ultimately embodied and grounded in iconicity and practical action rather than in genetically specified arbitrary codes. There are, however, two sources of evidence available from the archeological and historical records that support the idea that the development of language in the visual medium results, through a process of ritualization, in the codification and conventionalization of what begin as iconic signs for objects and their actions. Here we assume that languages are, in fact, human inventions and not merely automatic productions of a genetically based and directed drive to acquire language. Although we do not assume that a rigid bioprogram directs the development of individual languages, we do assert that there are constraints on the processes by which languages develop. In particular, we believe that human beings everywhere respond in similar ways to similar environmental and social pressures. It is this sort of general constraint or "canalization" of cultural development that gives rise to the similarities in the development of language in the visual medium that we will be discussing in this chapter. We will first consider what is known from the archeological record about the invention of

writing, and we will follow this with an account of what is known historically about the invention and development of signed languages—primarily
but not exclusively the signed languages of the deaf.

1 The Invention of Writing

The archeological record makes it clear that human beings do not begin to
write by first identifying and representing the elementary sound symbols
or phonemes of their languages. Instead, they tend generally first to create
visual representations that are relatively independent of their spoken languages. That is, the initial stages in the invention of writing seem to involve direct, pictorial representations of objects or numbers. According to
Givón,

> as in the case of sign language, the natural evolution of writing
> in all five centers where literacy is known to have arisen
> independently—China, India, Mesopotamia, Egypt, Maya—
> followed a similar course, from iconicity to abstraction. All five
> writing systems began with *iconic, pictorial* representation of a
> concrete lexicon. Their gradual move toward a more arbitrary
> code . . . came later. As elsewhere, the initial rise of a new code
> benefits from maximal iconicity. Only later does a code, rather
> inevitably, gravitate toward arbitrariness and symbolicity.
> (1998: 101)

Although it is perhaps only tangentially related to writing understood
as the visible representation on a surface of language existing originally in
some other medium, we begin this discussion with the oldest archeological evidence for human symbolic representation. This is widely accepted
to be the Paleolithic cave "art" of western Europe. Although we disagree
with this interpretation, we note that the appearance of this cave art, around
30,000 years ago, probably coincident with the arrival of *Homo sapiens* in
Europe, is sometimes taken as signaling the onset of full-fledged languages.
Some archaeologists have come to this conclusion simply because it is the
oldest evidence for human symbolic activity and, thus, the oldest evidence
of at least a capacity for symbolic representation, hence language. Of course,
we believe that true languages are much older than this. What we find most
interesting about this evidence is the fact that people around the world
who attain a level of technology generally labeled "Upper Paleolithic" tend
to produce these sorts of representations, and these representations tend
to have characteristics in common. Upper Paleolithic technologies can be
understood as advanced stone tool technologies in the absence of settled
agriculture; they are associated almost exclusively with *Homo sapiens* (and

perhaps very late Neanderthals); and they were characteristic of the entire human population of the world from perhaps 40,000 to about 10,000 years ago, when settled agricultural communities began to appear. These technologies persisted in parts of the world, primarily in the Americas, Australia, and parts of Africa, until virtually the present.

It is not known what the significance of this "art" may have been, but it is generally assumed that it had ritual purposes. The figures represented tend to be stylized pictures of animals and human beings. Stenciled outlines of hands are not uncommon. In figures 7.1 and 7.2, we present widely distributed examples from Europe (the Chauvet Cave, France, ca. 30,000 years B.P.) and North America. The obvious point is that stylized representations of objects important to human populations have a very long history, and there tend to be similarities in production that probably cannot be explained by cultural diffusion or sharing of ideas. These representations seem to involve something inherent in the process of human symbolic production.

There is a fascinating variation on the symbolism of this so-called rock art (as well as "artistic" representation in other media) from the native population of central Australia. Walbiri (or Warlpiri) nonfigurative art has been described as "discontinuous," meaning that it has discreet, iconic meaning units that can be recombined, and it has properties that are remi-

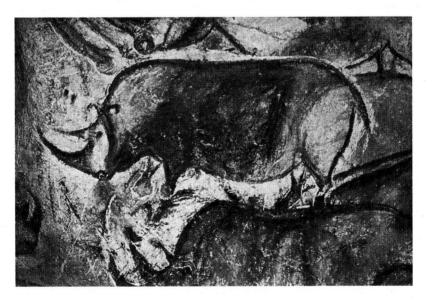

Figure 7.1. The most spectacular rhinoceroses in a group of seventeen. Representations of these animals are particularly plentiful in the Chauvet Cave. Photo by Jean Clottes. Courtesy of the Regional Directory of Cultural Affairs, Rhône-Alpes.

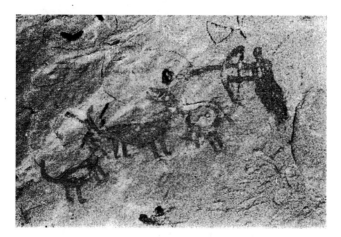

Figure 7.2. Three quadrupeds and hunter with bow and arrow. Native American petroglyph. Photo by Jay Crotty, Helen Crotty, and Ray Poore. Image courtesy of Chaco Culture National Historical Park, Albuquerque, New Mexico, Photo Archives, CHCU no. 43041.

niscent of the classifiers of signed languages that we discussed in chapter 3. In this system, patterns or shapes have distinctive meanings and can be used to represent a range of objects. For example, a circle might represent a water hole, a fruit, the base of tree, or a circular path; while a straight line might represent a straight path, the tail of a kangaroo, a spear, or a tree, and so on. Other shapes used in this way include curved lines and arches. Groups of dots might represent ants, and so on (Morwood, 2002: 95–96; Munn, 1973). This graphical notation system is used in body decoration, decoration of other objects, and in sand "painting" that accompanies narratives concerning the activities of ancestral beings. It is interesting that Walbiri (Warlpiri) women are one of a number of hearing Australian native populations that use a well-developed sign language, in addition to their spoken language (we discuss the worldwide distribution of similar systems later). Kendon (1988) has described this sign language. Descriptions of the use of this sign language in conjunction with the graphical system described earlier provide an insight into how writing systems might develop. In particular, women narrators may use both the sign language and the graphical system in storytelling:

> Both men and women draw similar graphic elements on the
> ground during storytelling or general discourse, but women
> formalize this narrative usage in a distinctive genre that I call a
> *sand story*. A space of about one to two feet in diameter is
> smoothed in the sand; the stubble is removed and small stones

plucked out. The process of narration consists of the rhythmic interplay of a continuous running graphic notation with gesture signs and a singsong verbal patter. The vocal accompaniment may sometimes drop to a minimum; the basic meaning is then carried by the combination of gestural and graphic signs. The gesture signs are intricate and specific and can substitute on occasion for a fuller verbalization. (Munn, 1973: 59–61)

Figure 7.3 illustrates some of the elements of a sand story.

Because this graphical notation system is fairly simple and restricted with respect to its elements, Kendon (1988: 433) describes it as "extra-linguistic" when seen in the context of the speech or sign language that it accompanies, but he may be underrating it. Munn (1973: 32) is explicit that because of its systematic use of "discontinuous" elements, the graphical system has some characteristics of a language. In fact, a similar set of graphical gestures used, apparently unconsciously, by military personnel in strategic discussions of maps has been described in the terms of signed language linguistics (Boudreau, 2003).

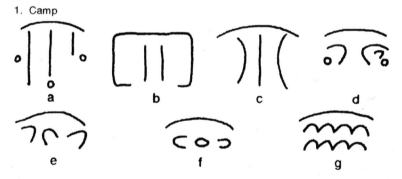

Figure 7.3. Elements of a Walbiri sand story. (a) Man, woman, and child sleeping in front of a bough shade; the woman is always beside the child (small line). O = fire. (b) A hut with two persons sleeping in it. The rectangular form is illustrated. (c) A man and two women (one on each side of him) sleeping in camp. This is a standard way of representing a man and two wives. (d) A man and woman sitting in camp are often shown facing in different directions. (The arc = bough shade.) A baby (small U shape) sits on the woman's lap. O = fire or food. (e) Three people sitting in camp. (f) Two people—e.g., man and wife—sitting in front of fire, eating. (g) Large number of persons sitting in men's or women's camps. From N. Munn, *Walbiri Iconography* (Ithaca, NY: Cornell University Press, 1973), 70. Reprinted with the permission of the author.

As was suggested in the quotation earlier, the development of writing seems to have followed similar paths in widely separated areas also. Although it has recently been claimed that there was a form of Inca writing involving a system of knot tying that was apparently entirely digital, perhaps without a prior form of pictographic writing (Mann, 2003), and that the first true writing, that of Sumer, was based on a system of clay tokens used in accountancy (Schmandt-Besserat, 1992—although some of these tokens were also clearly iconic), the general course of development of writing systems seems to follow that outlined in the earlier quotation by Givón. According to this formula, at some point in the evolution of technological and social complexity, a need arises for keeping more or less permanent records, and the first way of representing things in such records generally involves iconic, pictographic representations of objects, such as those shown in Sumerian pictograms (fig. 7.4).

Following this initial stage, written signs, logograms, come to represent words or morphemes, perhaps through some sort of evolution, perhaps through reinvention, with or without phonetic values also being assigned. At this stage, true writing of a spoken language has begun, as the words of the language start to be represented by individual signs.

The assignment of phonetic values seems to follow soon after the invention of logograms, and it generally seems to involve the discovery of what has been called the rebus principle. For example, in Egyptian hieroglyphic writing the iconic sign for the sun (Ra) comes to represent the syllable pronounced "ra," as in the phonetic representation of the name

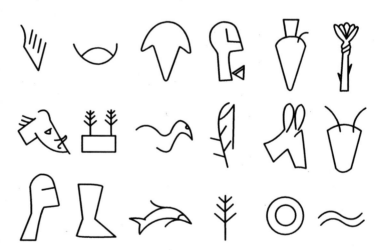

Figure 7.4. Sumerian pictograms. From Andrew Robinson, *Lost Languages: The Enigma of the World's Undeciphered Scripts* (New York: McGraw-Hill, 2002), page 25. Reprinted with permission of the McGraw-Hill Companies.

Ramses (see Robinson, 2002: 26). Thus, as scripts evolve further, they can come to incorporate more or less iconic logograms and phonetic elements. Here is an example of the homophonic rebus principle at work in the Mayan script (fig. 7.5):

> [This] is an affix often used as a locative preposition (such as "in" or "at" in English). It appears in a bewildering range of shapes: torches, bundles of sticks (usually smoking), wooden poles, a vulture head and others. The Maya treated them as equivalent signs, doubtless because the words for these objects were similar or identical to *ta,* the locative preposition in Cholan [a Mayan dialect]. The vulture was identified in Chol as *taʔ-hol,* "excrescence head," and the terms for pine and torch were *taaj.* (Houston, 1996: 37)

One final interesting point is that such logographic writing systems also tend to incorporate what are called "determinatives," nonphonetic classifiers that identify the semantic class of the logogram—for example, in Chinese writing, the class of objects made of wood. This can be compared to the classifiers of signed languages, described in previous chapters. Completely phonetic writing is rather rare as an independent invention, and its rarity is testimony to the nonobviousness of the phonemic structure of speech to most speakers.

Suggesting that there may be some sort of similar developmental progression of writing systems in widely separated parts of the world should in no way be taken as suggestive of the inherent superiority of a particular system, that is, the alphabet, or suggestive of some sort of evolutionary ranking. As with much else related to human difference, study of the evo-

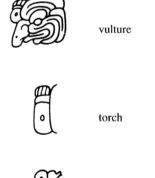

vulture

torch

bundle of pine

Figure 7.5. Homophonic Mayan glyphs. From Stephen D. Houston, *Reading the Past: Maya Glyphs* (Los Angeles: University of California Press, 1996), page 37. Reprinted with the permission of Stephen D. Houston and the Trustees of the British Museum.

lution of writing systems has an unsavory past influenced by European racism. According to many early accounts, writing systems like the Chinese were "ideographic," representing universal ideas and not the individual words of the language. This was perhaps influenced by the fact that, because Chinese logograms are relatively independent of the sound systems of Chinese languages, they were adopted and adapted by speakers of other languages, such as Japanese and Korean, to represent words with similar meanings in those languages. Europeans assumed that these signs were nonphonetic, hence less advanced than alphabetic systems. Chinese writing, of course, in addition to its logographic base, has a strong phonetic element, and it has effectively served one of the world's most complex civilizations for thousands of years. Nevertheless, prejudice against it and similar systems continues to linger. Failure by some scholars to believe that a non-Western people could independently invent a writing system that contained phonetic elements obstructed the deciphering of the Maya writing system for more than a century (see Coe, 1999). It is perhaps worth noting that scholars and educators wishing to denigrate the signed languages of the deaf have also smeared them with the same "ideographic" brush (e.g. Mykelbust, 1957: 241).

Most scripts that have been invented to represent the spoken languages of the world have maintained complex visual systems of representation and have not been reduced to simple one-for-one character-for-phoneme symbols. Coe (1999: 264) has the following to say about possible reasons for this, and we think this supports our central thesis concerning the importance of the visual element in linguistic expression:

> Now, the ancient Maya scribes could have written *everything* expressed in their language using only the [phonetic] syllabic signary—but they did not, any more than did the Japanese with their *kana* signs, or the Sumerians or Hittites with *their* syllabaries, or the Egyptians with their stock of consonantal signs. The logograms just had too much prestige to abolish. And why should they have done so? "One picture is worth a thousand words," as the saying goes, and Maya logograms, like their Egyptian equivalents, are often remarkably pictorial and thus more immediately informative than a series of abstract phonetic signs: for example, the Maya could, and sometimes did, write out *balam,* "jaguar," syllabically as *ba-la-m(a),* but by using a jaguar's head for *balam,* the scribe could get his word across in a more dramatic fashion.

Before leaving the ancient world of the Classic Maya, we should note that they did not distinguish between "writing" and "painting" in their language (Coe, 1999: 249)—thus, as is true with respect to many writing systems, writing was art. To complete this circle of thought, it is also worth noting that gestural analysis can be usefully applied to the study of writing, painting, and art in general. A whole school of Western art, exemplified by Jackson Pollock and Willem de Kooning, evolved under the rubric of "gesture painting," or "action painting," the painting being the record on canvas of an act of creation. The art theorist Rudolf Arnheim understood intuitively the embodied nature of the visual arts, and the deep connections between vision and the hand, when he asked, "If vision is an active grasp, what does it take hold of?" (1974: 43).

The point of this exercise, of course, is to show that the human invention of linguistic systems does not seem to proceed by a bottom-up process of synthesis, with the elementary phonological symbols being identified first and then assembled into ever larger units—syllables, words, sentences, and so on. Instead, it seems to proceed by a process of analysis, from relatively large, meaningful units to smaller units that are parsed out of gestalts, exactly what is predicted by Stokoe's semantic phonology. What human beings seem to notice first is that the objects and events around them can be represented by signs that have analogous relationships with the objects or events referred to. Again, visual representation can be expected to precede auditory representation because of the vastly greater possibility for iconic productivity in the visual medium. Semantic phonology suggests that the answer to Arnheim's question is "it takes hold of language."

Next, we will explore the stages through which emergent signed languages develop, but before leaving this topic, we must note that, as with much else we have discussed in this book, finding a linkage between gestural language origins and pictographic writing is not new. As early as the 1730s, William Warburton, the bishop of Gloucester, suggested that spoken languages had evolved from gestural "languages of action" as alphabetic writing had evolved from pictographic or hieroglyphic writing (see Rosenfeld, 2001: 38–39).

2 The Invention of Modern Sign Languages

There is abundant evidence that full-fledged sign languages emerge naturally among anatomically modern human populations when certain conditions are present. They appear to emerge naturally among deaf people and their hearing relatives and associates, but they also emerge among hearing people when environmental or social conditions make speech undesirable or impossible. Sign languages, or at least sign systems, are known to have arisen in hearing populations under the following conditions:

Among Christian monks living under a code of silence (Barakat, 1975)

As a specialized language of women among Australian Aborigines
(Kendon, 1988; Umiker-Sebeok & Sebeok, 1978)

As a lingua franca among North American Plains Indians (Umiker-
Sebeok & Sebeok, 1978)

Among sawmill workers in a noisy environment (Meissner &
Phillpot, 1975)

For use by hunters to avoid being heard by prey (Armstrong, 1999:
128–129)

Such systems, codes, or languages, in fact, appear to have been wide-
spread among pre-Neolithic societies, and this may be taken as further
evidence of their ancient lineage. The probability that substantial numbers of deaf people lived in these societies, especially older people who
had lost their hearing, cannot be discounted.

There is evidence for the emergence of sign systems among small
groups of deaf people and, especially in traditional societies in historical
times, the hearing people in the communities where these deaf people live.
The former systems have generally been referred to as "homesigns" (see,
e.g. Goldin-Meadow & Feldman, 1977), and they have been documented
in a variety of areas (e.g. Torigoe & Takei, 2002). When they are restricted
to use by a small number of deaf people, usually family members, and they
are not transmitted across generations, they appear to remain relatively
simple and syntactically impoverished. Such sign systems may not evolve
into fully "syntacticized" languages (e.g., Washabaugh, 1986).

In some cases, however, homesigns may expand beyond small groups
of family members to larger social groups, including hearing people, especially in simple or traditional societies. The most famous example of this
phenomenon is probably the case of the sign language that developed on
the island of Martha's Vineyard (Groce, 1985). The English settlers of the
Vineyard, who began arriving in the mid–seventeenth century, had a high
incidence of genetic deafness. Because this was a small, relatively closed
and inbred society, many families included deaf members, and an indig-
enous sign language developed that was apparently used by both the deaf
and hearing islanders. By the time it came to the attention of scholars in
the late twentieth century, the language had already died out, so not much
is known about its structure. It has been inferred, however, that it may have
had a significant influence on the development of ASL, as many deaf island children began to attend residential schools for the deaf on the main-
land, especially the American School for the Deaf in Hartford, Connecticut
(73). Comparable sign systems have been reported in use by deaf and hearing people among the Yucatec Maya of Mexico (Johnson, 1991) and on the
island of Bali (Branson, Miller, & Masaja, 1996). In his article on the Yucatec
Maya, Johnson also mentions unpublished reports of similar situations in
Venezuela, in Africa, and on the Navajo reservation in Arizona.

The true linguistic status of sign systems such as these may be difficult to determine, because they are seldom called on to carry the full weight of social commerce in the societies in which they exist—that is, they exist in parallel with spoken languages. However, there is no doubt that when deaf people live together in sufficient numbers, full-fledged sign languages emerge. How this might happen is illustrated by the emergence of three sign languages for which historical documentation exists: LSF, ASL, and NSL.

The earliest information that comes close to providing a linguistic description of a natural sign language has to do with LSF. French Sign Language is frequently said to have originated with the founding of the school for the deaf by the Abbé de l'Epée in Paris during the middle of the eighteenth century. It appears likely, however, that Epée drew on an existing sign language in formulating his system of "methodical" signs that were intended to support instruction in the written French language and that were grammatically modeled on that language. Little is known about natural sign languages that might have been in use by the French deaf community either before or immediately after the founding of Epée's school, but one source is what appears to be the first book ever published by a deaf author, Pierre Desloges's 1779 *Observations of a Deaf-Mute* (Fischer, 2002). Desloges made it clear in this book that there were grammatical differences between the French language and the sign language used by deaf people, especially with respect to the use of space, including the use of directional signs (Fischer, 2002).

Desloges also proposed a taxonomy of LSF signs. According to Fischer (2002), Desloges maintained that there are three classes of signs: "ordinary or primitive" signs, "reflected" signs, and "analytic" signs. As described, these are fairly familiar categories—the first comprises "natural signs which all peoples of the world, hearing or deaf, use frequently"—these are the largely iconic gestures of ordinary discourse that are incorporated into the sign language. The second category consists of signs that "can also be described as natural, but which can only be produced and understood with a certain amount of reflection." Finally, analytic signs stand "for concepts which are not suited for direct, pictorial expression." Desloges, thus, categorized the signs of this early form of LSF in terms of their relative iconicity.

The historical route whereby LSF came to influence the development of ASL is well known to the American deaf community and is worth recounting. This influence began with the arrival of Laurent Clerc in the United States to begin his partnership with Thomas Hopkins Gallaudet at the American School for the Deaf in Hartford in the early nineteenth century. Gallaudet brought Clerc, a deaf teacher, from France to begin the practice of teaching deaf children in sign language in the United States. Certainly, Clerc would at first have been teaching in LSF, but eventually a new language began to emerge, almost certainly incorporating elements of existing American sign systems, probably including the sign language of Martha's Vineyard. In commenting on the belief of Jean Marc Itard that LSF was highly iconic, Lane (1976: 235–236) outlines some of the processes that might have been at work, assuming, as many linguists do, that modern ASL is much less so:

> Perhaps . . . Franslan [LSF] was more iconic than Ameslan [ASL]. There are two reasons for thinking this. First, as signs are handed down from generation to generation, as the primary language of the family, from parent to child who becomes a parent in turn, they become simpler, more regular; they are shaped by the general rules for sign formation and thus become more encoded. Second, Franslan built originally on family signs brought to it by children like Massieu and his predecessors under Epée. De Gérando tells us that these children from isolated parts of France often brought similar signs for the same things.

Now ASL is the sign language that has been most thoroughly described and analyzed in linguistic terms, and this passage from Lane reflects a theoretical position that developed during the 1960s and 1970s to explain the obvious iconicity of ASL but nevertheless preserve its linguistic status. Early theory assumed that, while elements of the language might initially be introduced iconically, most iconicity was squeezed out over time by purely linguistic processes (Frishberg, 1975; Klima & Bellugi, 1979). Elsewhere (chapter 5) we have referred to this as attempting to banish the "specter" of iconicity, assumed to be necessary if the presumption is accepted that linguistic signs must be arbitrary. However, there are now linguistically sophisticated approaches to the description of ASL that assume not only that iconicity is involved at the beginnings of sign formation but also that it is basic to the ongoing grammatical processes of sign languages (Taub, 2001; P. Wilcox, 2000).

It is clear that much of the iconicity has also remained in the basic lexicons of signed languages, even following the evolutionary processes described earlier, and we believe that the reasons are even stronger than those that have led to the retention of iconic elements in many writing systems. Attempts have been made to estimate the iconic content of signed languages—for example, Pietrandrea's estimate (2002: 300) that 50 percent of the occurrences of handshapes in the lexicon of LIS are motivated by iconic associations and that 67 percent of the body locations are similarly motivated. Perusal of the dictionaries of as many signed languages as we could find convinces us that these percentages are not atypical. With respect to the overall iconicity of a particular signed language, however, simple counting of the iconic associations represented in a dictionary will tend toward underestimates, as the grammars of these languages also tend to be analogical to a high degree because, as we have pointed out elsewhere, of the extensive use of pointing and motivated classifier constructions. Recall also from the discussion in chapter 5 that Bouvet implies that virtually the entire lexicon of LSF can be shown, by working out its metaphoric basis, to have iconic associations. What is significant is that these languages could tend toward completely arbitrary codes and abstract grammatical processes if their users so desired—they just don't.

3 Origins of Sign Language: Emergent or Innate?

Direct evidence concerning the way sign languages originally emerge has recently come to light. The appearance of what is apparently a completely new sign language among deaf students in Nicaragua has focused linguists' attention on the factors that may be involved in the development of language in general, not just sign languages. In fact, the appearance of this language and the discussion surrounding its description has become a focal point in the ongoing debate about the modularity of language and the extent to which it represents a "faculty" separate in genetic determination from other human behavioral systems. The significance of this can be judged by the stature of the researchers and theorists who have become involved in the debate, including, according to a recent report in *Science* (Helmuth, 2001: 1758–1759): Steven Pinker, Lila Gleitman, Ann Senghas, and Dan Slobin. Pinker (1994: 36), citing Kegl (Kegl & Iwata, 1989), discusses the emergence of NSL as a key support for his "language as instinct" hypothesis:

> Until recently there were no sign languages at all in Nicaragua, because its deaf people remained isolated from one another. When the Sandinista government took over in 1979 and reformed the educational system, the first schools for the deaf were created. The schools focused on drilling the children in lip reading and speech, and as in every case where that is tried, the results were dismal. But it did not matter. On the playgrounds and schoolbuses, the children were inventing their own sign system, pooling the makeshift gestures that they used with their families at home.

In the popular press, the emergence of NSL into what now appears to be a full-fledged language, complete with complex syntax, has been taken as final proof of the Chomskyan hypothesis that human beings have a genetically determined "language organ" that always cranks out a language guided by principles of "universal grammar," whenever social conditions are minimally adequate (see, e.g., Osborne, 1999). At least the first part of this assertion is true with respect to sign languages—they always seem to emerge when speech is not feasible. What is in question is the second part of the assertion, the degree to which the details of the grammar are genetically determined, or stipulated.

For NSL to provide a pure "test case," it would be necessary for the deaf children of Nicaragua, before 1979, to have been completely cut off from human language. But how cut off were they? Certainly, as suggested in Pinker's account, they, like all other deaf people, had access to—at least idiosyncratic—homesigns. A recent historical account (Polich, 2000) suggests that the situation in which the language developed may have been quite complex, and may have included substantial contacts among homesigning deaf children prior to the early 1980s. According to Polich, there may also have been influences from foreign sign languages, including ASL and Costa Rican Sign Language. In the final analysis, however, the more fundamental question may be one that has arisen throughout this book.

Few would doubt that iconicity and indexicality are sources of sign language *signs*, but what is the source of the grammar of a new sign language like NSL? Does it arise because human brains are genetically predisposed to create certain kinds of grammatical structures or does it come from a more plastic brain that tends to solve similar problems in similar ways? This is a question that has been at the heart of a long-running debate in the science of language generally, and sign languages may provide a key to answering it, and thus answering the more general question of how all languages arise. Consider this quotation from Helmuth (2001: 1758), citing Senghas:

> She focused on a form of grammar common to every known
> sign language but absent from spoken languages. Signers use
> locations in space to show how objects or ideas are related. For
> instance, making the sign for "cup" in a certain spot, followed
> by the sign for "tall" in that spot, makes it clear that the cup—
> and not necessarily the person drinking from it—is tall.

Does this sort of strategy for using space, common to all sign languages, and now emerging, apparently independently, in NSL, represent a genetically encoded grammatical principle or does it reflect some "natural" need to communicate and simple efficiency in using the resources at hand? The final word is left to Stokoe (2000: 13). He comments here on a report about NSL signers that appeared in the *New York Times*:

> Their gestures naturally—not mysteriously or because of gram-
> mar rules—resemble or point at things and express actions with
> manual movement. For example, they sign "tell" by moving the
> hand from the teller to the one told. Kegl hails this as "verb
> agreement" and proof positive that, without any grammatical
> input, these children have invented grammar and language on

the spot. But signing "tell" as they do is hardly a strategy requiring grammar rules, universal or otherwise. After all, these children know as we all do that telling, like a Frisbee going from thrower to catcher, is action directed from one to another.

Whatever the role of outside influences may have been in the evolution of NSL, recent research on its development by Senghas, Kita, and Ozyurek (2004) provides much support for the scenario that we have presented here. Senghas and her colleagues examined three cohorts of Nicaraguan signers— essentially, first-, second-, and third-generation signers—and compared their signing to the gesturing accompanying the Spanish language speech of Nicaraguan hearing subjects. The logic of the experiment is that the signing of the older deaf signers should represent something like the language in its earliest stages, that of the second generation a more developed linguistic system, and so on. Senghas and colleagues elicited narratives from their subjects that involved verbal expressions of path and manner of motion, which, typically, are separately and sequentially encoded in spoken languages, as in "a ball rolls down a hill," but can be expressed simultaneously *or* sequentially in gesture or sign. Comparing the four groups of subjects— Spanish-speaking hearing gesturers and first-, second-, and third-generation signers, Senghas found that the hearing speakers never segmented their gestures for manner and path, for example when describing something rolling down a hill, that the first-generation signers infrequently segmented these gestures, and that the second- and third-generation signers frequently did.

The signs and gestures illustrated in the Senghas article appear quite iconic, and the authors make the following observation about their findings (Senghas, Kita, & Ozyurek, 2004: 1780–1781):

> In appearance, the signs very much resemble the gestures that accompany speech. The movements of the hands and body in the sign language are clearly derived from a gestural source. Nonetheless, the analyses reveal a qualitative difference between gesturing and signing. In gesture, manner and path were integrated by expressing them simultaneously and holistically, the way they occur in the motion itself. Despite this analog, holistic nature of the gesturing that surrounded them, the first cohort of children, who started building NSL in the late 1970s, evidently introduced the possibility of dissecting out manner and path and assembling them into a sequence of elemental units. As second and third cohorts learned the language in the mid-1980s and 1990s, they rapidly made this segmented, sequenced construction the preferred means of expressing motion events. NSL, thus, quickly acquired the discrete, combinatorial nature that is a hallmark of language.

We conclude this chapter by mentioning two additional cases of language emerging among deaf people. The first has been reported too recently for us to do a thorough analysis. It involves a small Bedouin village in the Negev desert of Israel in which, because of a genetic founder effect similar to that of Martha's Vineyard in the eighteenth and nineteenth centuries, a high proportion of deafness in the population has led to the emergence of a sign language in use by the deaf people of the village, as well as many of the hearing people. Again, as far as we can tell, this language has followed a course in which iconic gesture becomes conventionalized through use (Sandler et al., 2005), much like that described earlier for NSL.

Finally, in an analysis of the signing of three deaf Brazilians who were not members of an extensive deaf community, Fusellier-Souza questions the commonly held view that some critical mass of deaf signers, especially in an educational facility for deaf people, is necessary for language-like signing to emerge. She calls the signing done by these deaf people "Emerging Signed Languages" (ESLs). These appear to have been elaborated out of what we have elsewhere referred to as homesigns. Drawing on terminology introduced by Cuxac (2000), she (Fusellier-Souza, 2006) examines the signing of these deaf people sorted into two main tracks: "illustrative (or highly iconic) signing," and "stabilized gestural signs." This amounts, we believe, to a distinction between ad hoc illustration of events and a set of signs that have been conventionalized (through ritualization) between the deaf signers and the (primarily) hearing people with whom they interact. Fusellier-Souza writes:

> It appears from this analysis that an initial process of iconization of experience, evidenced in these languages, follows a structural course. The existence of gestural signs representing HIS [Highly Iconic Structures] and stabilized forms demonstrates that the bifurcation of the signers' intents into two structural branches ("telling while showing" or "telling without showing"), a process identified in the evolution of SLs used by deaf communities, is already at work in these three ESLs.
>
> I have observed that the illustrative branch permits these signers not only to construct a concept in an illustrative intent when they do not have a stabilized sign but also to elucidate, in a metalinguistic manner, a stabilized sign that has been topicalized in discourse. (46–48)

A plausible case can thus be made for the origin of signs and the rules that allow them to refer to relationships, and thus of sign *languages*, in the stuff of iconic and mimetic manual gesture. Given the information we have just considered, it is clear that the archeological and historical records support this conclusion. Finally, and most significantly, the origin of language itself, whether signed or spoken, can be traced to the same source.

Epilogue

A Vision of Unity

The British physicist Paul Davies once remarked that "all science is the search for unity" (Davies, 1984: 6). From the cosmologist's quest to see the birth of our universe in the glimmer of distant stars to the anthropologist's hunt for our hominid ancestors and the biologist's search for the origins of species, scientists search for that which unites the known with the unknown, the familiar with the unfamiliar, the present with the past.

One reason that scientists spend their lives in this pursuit is that unity offers at least partial explanations for phenomena not previously understood. As the physical anthropologist Matt Cartmill has noted, "to explain something is to show that it is an instance of some general rule, familiar to us from other instances" (1993: 226).

It is worth noting that the inverse situation—a unique phenomenon—does not merely pose a difficulty for science, it renders scientific explanation mute. Cartmill continues (1993: 226):

> If there really are human peculiarities that find no parallels in other creatures, then they are inexplicable. As long as we insist on hearing stories that "explain" human uniqueness, we will have to forgo genuine explanations and content ourselves with narrative fables, in which all the causal links are supplied by the imagination.

Another way to explain phenomena is to search for sources. In an essay on human uniqueness and the quest for the origins of language, Cartmill observes that

to understand the origin of anything, we must have an overarching body of theory that governs both the thing itself and its
precursors. Without such a body of theory, we have no way of
linking the precursor to its successors, and we are left with an
ineffable mystery, like the one that Chomsky and Lenneberg
have always insisted must lie at the origin of syntax. (1990: 188)

There are a number of ways scientists may search for sources and explanation in the study of language; as well, there are pitfalls to be avoided
if we are not to render science powerless by erecting unbreachable claims
of uniqueness. In this book we have argued that signed languages are in an
important sense not unique, that they are merely manifestations of the
human language ability, unfamiliar only because language scientists of the
time were not familiar with deaf people and their natural languages. This
in turn led to several questions: What is the precursor of human language?
Are signed languages implicated in the origin of language? What are the
precursors of signed language? Is there a link between sign and gesture?
Between gesture and language?

We have proposed that transformation of gesture into language lies
at the heart of the origin of language, that just as grammaticization-as-
ritualization accounts for the change from lexical to grammatical it also
accounts for the transformation of gesture into language. This reformu-
lation is compatible with the view that this "is part of the same [process]
as the transformation of actions into gestures, gestures into words, and
grammaticization in general" (Haiman, 1998b: 132). Haiman (1998a: 141)
concludes that this process "amounts to *the creation of (a) language out
of other kinds of behavior.*" Ritualization thus is implicated in the phylogenetic evolution of language from nonlinguistic behaviors, with visible gestures playing a key role.

Given the specter of the past when signed languages were denigrated
as "mere gesture," when powerful forces attempted to wipe them off the
face of the earth, and when deaf people were physically punished for using their natural languages, it is necessary to add a few final words about
what the search for the unification of gesture and sign language means,
and, more important, what it does not mean. Again, the words of Matt
Cartmill are exceptionally insightful. Writing of the backlash against teaching evolution in schools, he says (1998: 78):

You might think that by now everyone would have gotten used
to the idea that we are blood kin to all other organisms, and

closer kin to great apes than to spiders. On the face of it, the idea makes a certain amount of plain common sense. We all know that we share more features with apes than we do with spiders or snails or cypress trees. The theory of evolution simply reads those shared features as family resemblances. It doesn't deny that people are unique in important ways. Our kinship with apes doesn't mean we're only apes under the skin, any more than the kinship of cats with dogs means that your cat is repressing a secret urge to bark and bury bones.

We do not deny that we can find important differences between gestures and signs, and between gesture and language. Our attempt to unify gesture with language does not deny that signed languages are unique in important ways. Suggesting that signed languages are kin to gestures doesn't mean that signed languages are only gestures under the skin. It simply means we must recognize that the remarkable family resemblances between signs and gestures, and the tight integration of speech and gesture, imply a common ancestor.

At first glance (and as a final thought), it might seem a bit paradoxical that we have found a principle that unifies human spoken languages with the behavior of our primate relatives and ancestors by pursuing the implications of two simple observations—that vision is the master sense of the higher primates and that social living is their primary adaptation. From this comes the principle that examining visible gesture is the key to understanding the process by which communication among these animals became increasingly flexible and complex. It is the cultural (and to some extent the coevolved genetic) achievement of the human species to have discovered how to translate the power to represent the world visually into the economical and efficient modality of speech—and to get a glimpse of humans' visual/gestural past, one need only look at its vestiges in everyday behavior. We believe that the final proof of our thesis lies in the fact that those persons who cannot hear and speak, apparently without the need for instruction, readily return to the wellspring of all human language: signed language.

References

Allan, K. (1977). Classifiers. *Language,* 53(2), 285–311.

Arbib, M. A., & Rizzolatti, G. (1996). Neural expectations: A possible evolutionary path from manual skills to language. *Communication and Cognition,* 29(3–4), 393–424.

Armstrong, D. F. (1999). *Original signs: Gesture, sign and the sources of language.* Washington, DC: Gallaudet University Press.

Armstrong, D. F., & Katz, S. H. (1981). Brain laterality in signed and spoken language: A synthetic theory of language use. *Sign Language Studies,* 33, 319–350.

Armstrong, D. F., Stokoe, W. C., & Wilcox, S. E. (1995). *Gesture and the nature of language.* Cambridge: Cambridge University Press.

Armstrong, D. F., & Wilcox, S. (2003).Origins of sign language. In M. Marscharck & P. Spencer (Eds.), *Handbook of deaf studies, language, and education,* 305–318. New York: Oxford University Press.

Arnheim, R. (1974). *Art and visual perception: A psychology of the creative eye.* Berkeley: University of California Press.

Atkinson, J. (2000). *The developing visual brain.* Oxford: Oxford University Press.

Balter, M. (2002). "Speech gene" tied to modern humans. *Science,* 297, 1105.

Barakat, R. (1975). On ambiguity in Cistercian Sign Language. *Sign Language Studies,* 8, 275–289.

Battison, R. (1978). *Lexical borrowing in American Sign Language.* Silver Spring, MD: Linkstok Press.

Bauman, H-D. L. (2003). Rede*sign*ing literature: The cinematic poetics of American Sign Language poetry. *Sign Language Studies,* 4(1), 34–47.

Baynton, D. (2002). The curious death of sign language studies in the nineteenth century. In D. F. Armstrong, M. A. Karchmer, & J. V. Van Cleve (Eds.), *The study of signed languages: Essays in honor of William C. Stokoe*, 13–34. Washington, DC: Gallaudet University Press.

Begun, D. R. (1994). Relations among the great apes and humans: New interpretations based on the fossil record. *Yearbook of Physical Anthropology*, 37, 11–63.

Berger, P., & T. Luckmann. (1966). *The social construction of reality*. Garden City, NY: Doubleday.

Bickerton, D. (1990). *Language and species*. Chicago: University of Chicago Press.

Bickerton, D. (1995). *Language and human behavior*. Seattle: University of Washington Press.

Blake, J. (2000). *Routes to child language: Evolutionary and developmental precursors*. Cambridge: Cambridge University Press.

Blake, J., & Dolgoy, S. (1993). Gestural development and its relation to cognition during the transition to language. *Journal of Nonverbal Behavior*, 17, 87–102.

Blest, A. (1963). The concept of "ritualization." In W. Thorpe & O. Zangwill (Eds.), *Current problems in animal behavior*. Cambridge: Cambridge University Press.

Boesch, C. B., & H. Boesch-Achermann. (2000). *The chimpanzees of the Tai forest: Behavioural ecology and evolution*. Oxford: Oxford University Press.

Bolinger, D. (1983). Intonation and gesture. *American Speech*, 58(2), 156–174.

Bolinger, D. (1986). *Intonation and its parts: Melody in spoken English*. Stanford, CA: Stanford University Press.

Boudreau, G. (2003). Symbolic properties of graphical actions. *Sign Language Studies*, 4(1), 48–67.

Bouvet, D. (1997). *Le corps et la métaphore dans les langues gestuelles: A la recherche des modes de production des signes*. Paris: L'Harmattan.

Branson, J., Miller, D., & Masaja, I. J. (1996). Everyone here speaks sign language too: A deaf village in Bali, Indonesia. In C. Lucas (Ed.), *Multicultural aspects of sociolinguistics in deaf communities*, 39–57. Washington, DC: Gallaudet University Press.

Brouland, J. (1855). *Langage Mimique: Spécimen d'un dictionaire des signes*. Gallaudet Archives, Gallaudet University, Washington, DC.

Browman, C. P., & Goldstein, L. (1989). Articulatory gestures as phonological units. *Phonology*, 6, 201–251.

Burling, R. (1993). Primate calls, human language and nonverbal communication. *Current Anthropology*, 34(1), 25–53.

Burling, R. (1999). Motivation, conventionalization, and arbitrariness in the origin of language. In B. J. King (Ed.), *The origins of language: What nonhuman primates can tell us*, 307–350. Santa Fe, NM: School of American Research Press.

Bybee, J. L. (2003). Cognitive processes in grammaticization. In M. Tomasello (Ed.), *The new psychology of language: Cognitive and functional approaches to language structure*, Vol. 2, 145–167. Mahwah, NJ: Erlbaum.

Bybee, J., Perkins, R., & Pagliuca, W. (1994) *The evolution of grammar: tense, aspect, and modality in the languages of the world.* Chicago: University of Chicago Press.

Cagle, K. (2001). *One thousand ASL faces.* St. Louis, MO: Signs of Development.

Calbris, C. (1985). Space-time: Gestures as an expression of time; Espace-temps: Expression gestuelle du temps. *Semiotica,* 55, 1–2.

Calbris, G. (1990). *The semiotics of French gestures.* Bloomington: Indiana University Press.

Cantalupo, C., & Hopkins, W. D. (2001). Asymmetric Broca's area in great apes. *Nature,* 414, 505.

Capirci, O., Caselli, M. C., Iverson, J. M., Pizzuto, E., & Volterra, V. (2002). Gesture and the nature of language in infancy: The role of gesture as a transitional device en route to two-word speech. In D. F. Armstrong, M. A. Karchmer, & J. V. Van Cleve (Eds.), *The study of signed languages: Essays in honor of William C. Stokoe,* 213–246. Washington, DC: Gallaudet University Press.

Cartmill, M. (1990). Human uniqueness and theoretical content in paleo-anthropology. *International Journal of Primatology,* 11(3), 173–192.

Cartmill, M. (1993). *A view to a death in the morning: Hunting and nature through history.* Cambridge, MA: Harvard University Press.

Cartmill, M. (1998). Oppressed by evolution. *Discover,* 19(3), 78–83.

Chomsky, N. (1966). *Cartesian linguistics.* New York: Harper and Row.

Chomsky, N. (1972). *Language and mind.* New York: Harcourt Brace Jovanovich.

Coe, M. D. (1999). *Breaking the Maya code.* New York: Thames and Hudson.

Comrie, B. (1976). *Aspect: An introduction to the study of verbal aspect and related problems.* Cambridge: Cambridge University Press.

Corballis, M. C. (2002). *From hand to mouth: The origins of language.* Princeton, NJ: Princeton University Press.

Corballis, M. C. (2003). From mouth to hand: Gesture, speech, and the evolution of right-handedness. *Behavioral and Brain Sciences,* 26(2), 199–208

Croft, W., & Cruse, D. A. (2004). *Cognitive linguistics.* Cambridge: Cambridge University Press.

Cuxac, C. (2000). *La Langue des Signes Française: Les Voies de l'Iconicité.* Faits de Langues no. 15–16. Paris: Ophrys.

Davies, P. (1984). *Superforce.* New York: Simon and Schuster.

Deacon, T. (1997). *The symbolic species: The co-evolution of language and the brain.* New York: Norton.

Deane, P. D. (1992). *Grammar in mind and brain: Explorations in cognitive syntax.* Berlin: de Gruyter.

de Jorio, A. (2000 [1832]). *Gesture in Naples and gesture in classical antiquity* (Adam Kendon, Trans. and Ed.). Bloomington: Indiana University Press.

DeMatteo, A. (1977). Visual imagery and visual analogues in ASL. In L. A. Friedman (Ed.), *On the other hand,* 109–136. New York: Academic Press.

Descartes, R. (1980 [1641]). *Discourse on method and meditations on first philosophy* (D. A. Cress, Trans.). Indianapolis: Hackett.

Duncan, S. (2002). Gesture, verb aspect, and the nature of iconic imagery in natural discourse. *Gesture,* 2(2), 183–206.

Emmorey, K. (2002). *Language, cognition, and the brain: Insights from sign language research.* Mahwah, NJ: Erlbaum.

Emmorey, K., & Riley, J. (Eds.). (1995). *Sign, gesture, and space.* Hillsdale, NJ: Erlbaum.

Enard, W., Przeworski, M., Fisher, S. E., Lai, C. S. L., Wiebe, V., Kitano, T., Monaco, A. P., & Paabo, S. (2002). Molecular evolution of FOXP2, a gene involved in speech and language, *Nature, 418,* 869–872.

Engberg-Pedersen, E. (1993). *Space in Danish Sign Language: The semantics and morphosyntax of the use of space in a visual language.* Hamburg: SIGNUM-Verlag.

Fauconnier, G. (1985). *Mental spaces.* Cambridge, MA: MIT Press.

Fauconnier, G. (1997). *Mappings in thought and language.* New York: Cambridge University Press.

Fauconnier, G., & Turner, M. (1996). Blending as a central process of grammar. In A. E. Goldberg (Ed.), *Conceptual structure, discourse, and language,* 113–130. Stanford, CA: Center for the Study of Language and Information Publications.

Fauconnier, G., & Turner, M. (2002). *The way we think: Conceptual blending and the mind's hidden complexities.* New York: Basic Books.

Fischer, R. (2002). The study of natural sign language in eighteenth-century France. *Sign Language Studies, 2*(4), 391–406.

Fisher, S. E., Vargha-Kadem, F., Watkins, K. E., Monaco, A. P., & Pembrey, M. E. (1998). Localisation of a gene implicated in a severe speech and land language disorder. *Nature Genetics, 18,* 168–170.

Fitch, W. T., & Hauser, M. D. (2004). Computation constraints on syntactic processing in a nonhuman primate. *Science, 303*(5656), 377–80.

Fouts, R., & Mills, S.T. (1997). *Next of kin.* New York: Morrow.

Frishberg, N. (1975). Arbitrariness and iconicity: Historical change in American Sign Language. *Language, 51,* 699–719.

Fusellier-Souza, I. (2006). Emergence and development of signed languages: From a semiogenetic point of view. *Sign Language Studies, 7*(1), 30–56.

Gallaudet, E. M. (1983). *History of the college for the deaf, 1857–1907.* Washington, DC: Gallaudet College Press.

Gannon, P. J., Holloway, R. L., Broadfield, D.C., & Braun, A. R. (1998). Asymmetry of chimpanzee planum temporale: Human-like brain pattern of Wernicke's area homolog. *Science, 279,* 220–221.

Gärdenfors, P. (2004). *Conceptual spaces: The geometry of thought.* Cambridge, MA: MIT Press.

Gardner, R. E., Gardner, B. T., & Van Canfort, T. E. (1989). *Teaching sign language to chimpanzees.* Albany: State University of New York Press.

Gelernter, D. (1998). *Machine beauty: Elegance and the heart of technology.* New York: Basic Books.

Ghazanfar, A. A., & Logothetis, N. K. (2003). Facial expressions linked to monkey calls. *Nature, 423,* 937–938.

Gibbons, A. (2006). *The first human: The race to discover our earliest ancestors.* New York: Doubleday.

Gibson, K. R. (1997). Review of *The wisdom of the bones* by A. Walker and P. Shipman. *Evolution of Communication, 1*(1), 153–155.

Gibson, K. R., & Jesse, S. (1999). Language evolution and expansion of multiple neurological processing areas. In B. J. King (Ed.), *The origins of language: What nonhuman primates can tell us*, 189–227. Santa Fe, NM: School of American Research Press.

Givens, D. B. (1986). The big and the small: Toward a paleontology of gesture. *Sign Language Studies*, 51, 145–170.

Givón, T. (1989). *Mind, code and context: Essays in pragmatics*. Hillsdale, NJ: Erlbaum.

Givón, T. (1995). *Functionalism and grammar*. Amsterdam: John Benjamins.

Givón, T. (1998). On the co-evolution of language, mind, and brain. *Evolution of Communication*, 2(1), 45–116.

Goldin-Meadow, S., & Feldman, H. (1977). The development of language-like communication without a language model. *Science*, 197, 401–403.

Goldin-Meadow, S., & Mylander, C. (1998). Spontaneous sign systems created by deaf children in two cultures. *Nature*, 391, 279–281.

Gómez, J. C. (1997). The study of the evolution of communication as a meeting of disciplines. *Evolution of Communication*, 1, 101–132.

Gopnick, M. (1990). Feature-blind grammar and dysphasia. *Nature*, 344, 715.

Groce, N. E. (1985). *Everyone here spoke sign language: Hereditary deafness on Martha's Vineyard*. Cambridge, MA: Harvard University Press.

Haiman, J. (1980). The iconicity of grammar: Isomorphism and motivation. *Language*, 56(3), 515–540.

Haiman, J. (1985). *Natural syntax*. Cambridge: Cambridge University Press.

Haiman, J. (1994). Ritualization and the development of language. In W. Pagliuca (Ed.), *Perspectives on grammaticalization*, 3–28. Amsterdam: John Benjamins.

Haiman, J. (1998a). The metalinguistics of ordinary language. *Evolution of Communucation*, 2(1), 117–135.

Haiman, J. (1998b). *Talk is cheap: Sarcasm, alienation, and the evolution of language*. Oxford: Oxford University Press.

Harnad, S. R., Steklis, H. D., & Lancaster, J. (Eds.). (1976). Origins and evolution of language and speech. [Special issue]. *Annals of the New York Academy of Sciences*, 280.

Harris, R. A. (1993). *The linguistics wars*. Oxford: Oxford University Press.

Hauser, M. D. (1996). *The evolution of communication*. Cambridge, MA: MIT Press.

Hauser, M. D., Chomsky, C., & Fitch, W. T. (2002). The faculty of language: What is it, who has it, and how did it evolve? *Science*, 298, 1569–1578.

Hayes, K.J., & Nissen, C. H. (1971). Higher mental functions of a home-raised chimpanzee. In A. M. Schrier & F. Stollnitz (Eds.), *Behavior of Non-Human Primates*, 59–115. New York: Academic Press.

Helmuth, L. (2001). From the mouths (and hands) of babes. *Science*, 293, 1758–1759.

Hewes, G. W. (1973). Primate communication and the gestural origin of language. *Current Anthropology*, 14, 5–24.

Hewes, G. W. (1976). The current status of the gestural theory of language origins. *Annals of the New York Academy of Sciences*, 280, 482–504.

Hewes, G. W. (1992). Primate communication and the gestural origin of language. *Current Anthropology*, 33 (supp.), 65–84.

Hewes, G. W. (1996). A history of the study of language origins and the gestural primacy hypothesis. In A. Lock and C. R. Peters (Eds.), *Handbook of human symbolic evolution*, 571–595. Oxford: Clarendon Press.

Higgins, D. D. (1923). *How to talk to the deaf.* St. Louis: Author.

Hockett, C. (1982). The origin of speech. In W. S.-Y. Wang (Ed.), *Human communication: Language and its psychobiological bases*, 5–12. San Francisco: Freeman.

Hockett, C. (1978). In search of Jove's brow. *American Speech*, 53, 243–315.

Holloway, R. L. (1983). Human paleontological evidence relevant to language behavior. *Human Neurobiology*, 2, 105–114.

Hopper, P. J. (1987). Emergent grammar. In *Papers of the Thirteenth Annual Meeting, Berkeley Linguistics Society*, 139–157. Berkeley: Berkeley Linguistics Society.

Hopper, P. (1994). Phonogenesis. In W. Pagliuca (Ed.), *Perspectives on grammaticization*, 29–45. Amsterdam: John Benjamins.

Hopper, P. J., & Thompson, S. A. (1984). The discourse basis for lexical categories in universal grammar. *Language*, 60(4), 703–52.

Houston, S. D. (1996). *Reading the past: Maya glyphs.* Los Angeles: University of California Press.

Hymes, D. (1971). Foreword to M. Swadesh, *The origin and diversification of language*, v–x. Chicago: Aldine.

Inoue-Nakamura, N., & Matsuzawa, T. (1997). Development of stone tool use by wild chimpanzees (pan Troglodytes). *Journal of Comparative Psychology*, 111(2), 159–173.

Iverson, J. M. (1998). Gesture when there is no visual model. *New Directions for Child Language*, 79, 89–100.

Jackendoff, R. (2002). *Foundations of language: Brain, meaning, grammar, evolution.* Oxford: Oxford University Press.

Jackendoff, R. (2003). *Precis of Foundations of language: Brain, meaning, grammar, evolution. Behavioral and Brain Sciences*, 26(6), 651–665.

Janzen, T. (2004). Space rotation, perspective shift, and verb morphology in ASL. *Cognitive Linguistics*, 15 (2), 149–174.

Janzen, T., & Shaffer, B. (2002). Gesture as the substrate in the process of ASL grammaticization. In R. Meier, D. Quinto, & K. Cormier (Eds.), *Modality and structure in signed and spoken languages*, 199–223. Cambridge: Cambridge University Press.

Janzen, T., Shaffer, B., & Wilcox, S. (2000). Signed language pragmatics. In J. Verschueren, J.-O. Östman, J. Blommaert, & C. Bulcaen (Eds.), *Handbook of Pragmatics*, 1–20. Amsterdam: John Benjamins.

Johnson, M. (1987). *The body in the mind: The bodily basis of meaning, imagination, and reason.* Chicago: University of Chicago Press.

Johnson, R. E. (1991). Sign language, culture, and community in a traditional Yucatec Maya village. *Sign Language Studies*, 73, 461–74.

Jowett, B. (1901). *The dialogues of Plato.* Vol. 1. New York: Scribner's.

Kegl, J., & Iwata, G. A. (1989). Lenguage de Signos Nicaragüense: A pidgin sheds light on the "creole"? In *Proceedings of the fourth annual meeting of the Pacific Linguistics Conference.* Eugene: University of Oregon.

Kelso, J. A. M., Saltzman, E. L., & Tuller, B. (1986). The dynamical perspective on speech production: Data and theory. *Journal of Phonetics*, 14, 29–59.

Kendon, A. (1980). Gesticulation and speech: Two aspects of the process of utterance. In M. R. Key (Ed.), *The relationship of verbal and nonverbal communication*, 207–228. The Hague: Mouton.

Kendon, A. (1988). *Sign languages of aboriginal Australia*. Cambridge: Cambridge University Press.

Kendon, A. (1991). Some considerations for a theory of language origins. *Man*, 26, 199–221.

Kendon, A. (1995). Gestures as illocutionary and discourse structure markers in Southern Italian conversation. *Journal of Pragmatics*, 23(3), 247–279.

Kendon, A. (2002). Historical observations on the relationship between research on sign languages and language origins theory. In D. F. Armstrong, M. A. Karchmer, & J. V. Van Cleve (Eds.), *The study of signed languages: Essays in honor of William C. Stokoe*, 13–34. Washington, DC: Gallaudet University Press.

Kimura, D. (1993). *Neuromotor mechanisms in human communication*. Oxford: Oxford University Press.

King, B. J. (1994). *The information continuum: Evolution of social information transfer in monkeys, apes, and hominids*. Santa Fe, NM: School of American Research Press.

King, B. J. (1999). Viewed from up close: Monkeys, apes, and language-origins theories. In B. J. King (Ed.), *The origins of language: What nonhuman primates can tell us*, 21–54. Santa Fe, NM: School of American Research Press.

King, B. J. (2003). Alternative pathways for the evolution of gesture [Review of *From Hand to mouth* by M. C. Corballis]. Sign Language Studies, 4(1), 68–82.

King, B. J. (2004). *The dynamic dance: Nonvocal communication in African great apes*. Cambridge, MA: Harvard University Press.

Klima, E., & Bellugi, U. (1979). *The signs of language*. Cambridge, MA: Harvard University Press.

Kluckhohn, C., & Leighton, D. (1951). *The Navaho*. Cambridge, MA: Harvard University Press.

Kövecses, Z. (2002). *Metaphor: A practical introduction*. New York: Oxford University Press.

Krebs, J. R., & Davies, N. B. (1993). *An introduction to behavioural ecology*. Oxford: Blackwell Science.

Lai, C. S., Fisher, S. E., Hurst, J. A., Vargha-Khadem, F., & Monaco, A. P. (2001). A forkhead-domain gene is mutated in a severe speech and language disorder. *Nature*, 413, 519.

Lakoff, G. (1987). *Women, fire, and dangerous things: What categories reveal about the mind*. Chicago: University of Chicago Press.

Lane, H. (1976). *The wild boy of Aveyron*. Cambridge, MA: Harvard University Press.

Lane, H. (1984). *When the mind hears*. New York: Random House.

Lang, H. (2003). Perspectives on the history of deaf education. In M. Marschark & P. E. Spencer (Eds.), *Oxford handbook of deaf studies, language, and education*, 9–20. New York: Oxford University Press.

Langacker, R. W. (1987). *Foundations of cognitive grammar. Vol. 1: Theoretical prerequisites*. Palo Alto, CA: Stanford University Press.

Langacker, R. W. (1988). An overview of cognitive grammar. In B. Rudzka-Ostyn (Ed.), *Topics in cognitive linguistics*, 3–48. Amsterdam: John Benjamins.

Langacker, R. W. (1991a). *Foundations of cognitive grammar. Vol. 2: Descriptive application*. Stanford, CA: Stanford University Press.

Langacker, R. W. (1991b). *Concept, image, and symbol: The cognitive basis of grammar*. Berlin: de Gruyter.

Langacker, R. W. (2000). *Grammar and conceptualization*. Berlin: de Gruyter.

Laughlin, C. D., & D'Aquli, E. G. (1974). *Biogenetic structuralism*. New York: Columbia University Press.

Leavens, D. A., Hopkins, W. D., & Bard, K. A. (1996). Indexical and referential pointing in chimpanzees (*Pan troglodytes*). *Journal of Comparative Psychology*, 110, 346–353.

Liddell, S. K. (1998). Grounded blends, gestures, and conceptual shifts. *Cognitive Linguistics*, 9(3), 283–314.

Liddell, S. K. (2002). Modality effects and conflicting agendas. In D. F. Armstrong, M. A. Karchmer, & J. V. Van Cleve (Eds.), *The study of signed languages: Essays in honor of William C. Stokoe*, 53–81. Washington, DC: Gallaudet University Press.

Liddell, S. K. (2003). *Grammar, gesture, and meaning in American Sign Language*. Cambridge: Cambridge University Press.

Liddell, S. K., & Johnson, R. E. (1989). American Sign Language: The phonological base. *Sign Language Studies*, 64, 195–277.

Liddell, S. K., & Metzger, M. (1998). Gesture in sign language discourse. *Journal of Pragmatics*, 30(6), 657–697.

Lieberman, P. (1991). *Uniquely human*. Cambridge, MA: Harvard University Press.

Lindblom, B. (1990). On the communication process: Speaker-listener interaction and the development of speech. In K. Fraurud & U. Sundberg (Eds.), *AAC augmentative and alternative communication*, 220–230. London: Williams and Wilkins.

McDonald, B. H. (1982). Aspects of the American Sign Language predicate system. Ph.D. diss., University of Buffalo.

McGurk, H., & MacDonald, J. (1976). Hearing lips and seeing voices. *Nature*, 264, 746–748.

McNeill, D. (1992). *Hand and mind: What gestures reveal about thought*. Chicago: University of Chicago Press.

Mann, C. C. (2003). Cracking the Khipu Code. *Science*, 300, 1650–1651.

Manning, A. (1967). *An introduction to animal behavior*. New York: Addison-Wesley.

Marzke, M. W. (1996). Evolution of the hand and bipedality. In A. Lock & C. R. Peters (Eds.), *Handbook of human symbolic evolution*, 126–154. Oxford: Clarendon Press.

Mead, G. H. (1970). *Mind, self, and society.* Edited and with an introduction by C. W. Morris. Chicago: University of Chicago Press. Originally published 1934.

Meier, R. P. (1991). Language acquisition by deaf children. *American Scientist,* 79, 60–70.

Meillet, A. (1948). *L'évolution des formes grammaticales.* Paris: Champion. Originally published in Science (Milan), 12(26) (1912).

Meissner, M., & Phillpott, S. (1975). The sign language of sawmill workers in British Columbia. *Sign Language Studies,* 9, 291–308.

Mitani, J. C., & Gros-Louis, J. (1998). Chorusing and call convergence in chimpanzees: Test of three hypotheses. *Behaviour,* 135, 1041–1064.

Morford, J. P., & Kegl, J. (2000). Gestural precursors to linguistic constructs: How input shapes the form of language. In D. McNeill (Ed.), *Language and gesture.* Cambridge: Cambridge University Press.

Morris, D., Collett, P., Marsh, P., & O'Shaughnessy, M. (1979). *Gestures: Their origin and distribution.* New York: Stein and Day.

Morwood, M. J. (2002). *Visions from the past: The archaeology of Australian Aboriginal art.* Washington, DC: Smithsonian Institution Press.

Munn, N. (1973). *Walbiri iconography.* Ithaca, NY: Cornell University Press.

Myers, R. (1976). Comparative neurology of vocalization and speech: Proof of a dichotomy. In S. Steklis, H. Harnad, & J. Lancaster (Eds.), Origins and evolution of language and speech (Special issue), *Annals of the New York Academy of Sciences,* 280, 745–757.

Myklebust, H. (1957). *The psychology of deafness.* New York: Grune and Stratton.

Napier, J. R., & Napier, P. H. (1967). *A handbook of living primates: Morphology, ecology and behaviour of nonhuman primates.* New York: Academic Press.

Neisser, U. (1967). *Cognitive psychology.* New York: Appleton-Century-Crofts.

Newport, E. L., & Meier, R. (1985). The acquisition of American Sign Language. In D. I. Slobin (Ed.), *The crosslinguistic study of language acquisition* (1: *The data*), 881–938. Hillsdale, NJ: Erlbaum.

Osborne, L. (1999). A linguistic big bang. *New York Times Magazine,* October 24, 84–89.

Parrill, F. (2000). Hand to mouth: Linking spontaneous gesture and aspect. Unpublished paper, Department of Linguistics, University of California, Berkeley.

Parrill, F. (2001). Linguistic aspect and gestural cues to backstage cognition. Paper presented at seventh International Cognitive Linguistics Conference, Santa Barbara, CA, July 22–27.

Peirce, C. S. (1955 [1940]). Logic as semiotic: The theory of signs. In J. Buchler (Ed.), *The philosophical writings of Peirce,* 98–119. New York: Dover.

Pennisi, E. (2006). Mining the molecules that made our mind. *Science,* 313, 1908–1911.

Petitto, L. A., Zatorre, R. J., Gauna, K., Nikelski, E. J., Dostie, D., & Evans, A. C. (2000). Speech-like cerebral activity in profoundly deaf people while processing signed languages: Implications for the neural basis of all human language. *Proceedings of the National Academy of Sciences,* 97(25), 13961–13966.

Pietrandrea, P. (2002). Iconicity and arbitrariness in Italian Sign Language. *Sign Language Studies*, 2(3), 296–321.

Pinker, S. (1994). *The language instinct.* New York: Morrow.

Plooij, Frans X. (1984). *The behavioral development of free-living chimpanzee babies and infants.* Norwood, NJ: Ablex.

Polich, L. (2000). The search for Proto-NSL: Looking for the roots of the Nicaraguan deaf community. In M. Metzger (Ed.), *Bilingualism and identity in deaf communities*, 255–305. Washington, DC: Gallaudet University Press.

Premack, D. (2004). Is language the key to human intelligence? *Science*, 303, 318–320.

Richmond, B. G., & Strait, D. S. (2000). Evidence that humans evolved from a knuckle-walking ancestor. *Nature*, 404, 382–385.

Rizzolatti, G., & Arbib, M. A. (1998). Language within our grasp. *Trends in Neuroscience*, 21, 188–194.

Rizzolatti, G., Fogassi, L., & Gallese, V. (1997). Parietal cortex: From sight to action. *Current Opinion in Neurobiology*, 7, 562–567.

Robinson, A. (2002). *Lost languages: The enigma of the world's undeciphered scripts.* New York: McGraw-Hill.

Rosenfeld, S. (2001). *A revolution in language: The problem of signs in late eighteenth-century France.* Stanford, CA: Stanford University Press.

Sandler, W., Meir, I., Padden, C., & Aronoff, M. (2005). The emergence of grammar: Systematic structure in a new language. *Proceedings of the National Academy of Sciences*, 102(7), 2661–2665.

Sapir, E. (1921) *Language.* New York: Harcourt, Brace, and World.

Savage-Rumbaugh, S. (1999). Ape language. In B. J. King (Ed.), *The origins of language: What nonhuman primates can tell us*, 115–188. Santa Fe, NM: School of American Research Press.

Schick, B. (2003). The development of American Sign Language and manually coded English systems. In M. Marschark & P. E. Spencer (Eds.), *Oxford handbook of deaf studies, language, and education*, 219–231. New York: Oxford University Press.

Schmandt-Besserat, D. (1992). *Before writing.* Austin: University of Texas Press.

Senghas, A., Kita, S., & Ozyurek, A. (2004). Children creating core properties of language: Evidence from an emerging sign language in Nicaragua. *Science*, 305, 1779–1782.

Sereno, M. I. (1991a). Four analogies between biological and cultural/linguistic evolution. *Journal of Theoretical Biology*, 151, 467–507.

Sereno, M. I. (1991b). Language and the primate brain. In *Proceedings of the Thirteenth Annual Cognitive Science Conference*, 79–84. Hillsdale, NJ: Erlbaum.

Shaffer, B. (2000). A syntactic, pragmatic analysis of the expression of necessity and possibility in American Sign Language. Ph.D. diss., University of New Mexico, Albuquerque.

Shaffer, B., & Janzen, T. (2000). Gesture, lexical words, and grammar: Grammaticization processes in ASL. Paper presented at the twenty-sixth annual meeting of the Berkeley Linguistics Society, Berkeley, CA, February 18–21.

Shanker, S., & King, B. J. (2002). The emergence of a new paradigm in ape language research. *Behavioral and Brain Sciences*, 25, 605–626.

Singleton, J. L., Morford, J. P., & Goldin-Meadow, S. (1993). Once is not enough: Standards of well-formedness in manual communication created over three different timespans. *Language*, 69(4), 683–715.

Steklis, H. (1985). Primate communication, comparative neurology, and the origin of language reexamined. *Journal of Human Evolution*, 14, 157–173.

Stokoe, W. C. (1960). *Sign language structure: An outline of the visual communication systems of the American deaf.* Studies in Linguistics, Occasional papers 8. Buffalo, NY: University of Buffalo Department of Anthropology and Linguistics.

Stokoe, W. C. (1976). Sign language autonomy. *Annals of the New York Academy of Sciences*, 280, 505–513.

Stokoe, W. C. (1980). Sign language structure. *Annual Review of Anthropology*, 9, 365–90.

Stokoe, W. C. (1991). Semantic phonology. *Sign Language Studies*, 71, 99–106.

Stokoe, W. C. (2000). Models, signs, and universal rules. *Sign Language Studies*, 1(1), 10–16.

Stokoe, W. C. (2001). *Language in hand: Why sign came before speech.* Washington, DC: Gallaudet University Press.

Stokoe, W. C., Casterline, D. C., & Croneberg, C. G. (1965). A *dictionary of American Sign Language on linguistic principles.* Washington, DC: Gallaudet College Press.

Studdert-Kennedy, M. (1987). The phoneme as a perceptuomotor structure. In D. A. Allport (Ed.), *Language perception and production: Relationships between listening, speaking, reading, and writing*, 67–84. London: Academic Press.

Supalla, T., & Newport, E. L. (1978). How many seats in a chair? In P. Siple (Ed.), *Understanding language through sign language research*, 91–132. New York: Academic Press.

Swadesh, M. (1971). *The origin and diversification of language.* Chicago: Aldine.

Tanner, J. E., & Byrne, R. W. (1996). Representation of action through iconic gesture in a captive lowland gorilla. *Current Anthropology*, 37, 12–73.

Tattersall, I. (1999). *Becoming human: Evolution and human uniqueness.* New York: Harcourt, Brace.

Taub, S. (2001). *Language from the body: Iconicity and metaphor in American Sign Language.* Cambridge: Cambridge University Press.

Taylor, T. (1996). The origin of language: Why it never happened. *Language Science*, 19, 67–77.

Tomasello, M. (1998). *The new psychology of language: Cognitive and functional approaches to language structure.* Mahwah, NJ: Erlbaum.

Tomasello, M., Call, J., Warren, J., Frost, G. T., Carpenter, M., & Nagell, K. (1997). The ontogeny of chimpanzee gestural signals: A comparison across groups and generations. *Evolution of Communication*, 1(2), 223–260.

Torigoe, T., & Takei, W. (2002). A descriptive analysis of pointing and oral movements in a homesign. *Sign Language Studies*, 2(3), 281–295.

Traugott, E. C. (1989). On the rise of epistemic meanings in English: An example of subjectification in semantic change. *Language*, 65(1), 31–55.

Tylor, E. B. (1865). *Researches into the early history of mankind and the development of civilization.* London: John Murray.

Umiker-Sebeok, D., & Sebeok, T. (1978). *Aboriginal sign languages of the Americas and Australia.* New York: Plenum Press.

Valli, C., & Lucas, C. (1995). *Linguistics of American Sign Language: An introduction.* Washington, DC: Gallaudet University Press.

van Lawick-Goodall, J. (1976). *In the shadow of man.* Boston: Houghton-Mifflin.

Veà, J. J., & Sabater-Pi, J. (1998). Spontaneous pointing in behaviour in the wild pygmy chimpanzee (*Pan paniscus*). *Folia Primatologica,* 69, 289–90.

Vygotsky, L. S. (1978). *Mind in society: The development of higher psychological processes.* Edited by M. Cole, V. John-Steiner, S. Scribner, & E. Souberman. Cambridge, MA: Harvard University Press.

Walker, A., & Shipman, P. (1996). *The wisdom of the bones: In search of human origins.* New York: Random House.

Wallman, J. (1992). *Aping language.* Cambridge: Cambridge University Press.

Washabaugh, W. (1986). *Five fingers for survival.* Ann Arbor, MI: Karoma.

Wescott, R. (Ed.). (1974). *Language origins.* Silver Spring, MD: Linstok Press.

Wilbur, R. (1987). *American Sign Language: Linguistic and applied dimensions.* Boston: Little Brown.

Wilcox, P. P. (2000). *Metaphor in American Sign Language.* Washington, DC: Gallaudet University Press.

Wilcox, S. (1993). Language from the body: Iconicity in signed languages. Paper presented at third conference of the International Cognitive Linguistics Association. Leuven, Belgium, July 18–23, 1993.

Wilcox, S. (1998). Cognitive iconicity and signed language universals. Paper presented at Cognitive Morphology Workshop, Ghent, Belgium, July 1–4, 1998.

Wilcox, S. (2000). *Gesture, icon, and symbol: The expression of modality in signed languages.* Paper presented at the twenty-sixth annual meeting of the Berkeley Linguistics Society, Berkeley, CA, February 18–21.

Wilcox, S. (2001). Conceptual spaces and bodily actions. Paper presented at seventh international conference of the International Cognitive Linguistics Association, Santa Barbara, CA, July 22–27.

Wilcox, S. (2002). The iconic mapping of space and time in signed languages. In L. Albertazzi (Ed.), *Unfolding perceptual continua,* 255–281. Amsterdam: John Benjamins.

Wilcox, S. (2004a). Cognitive iconicity: Conceptual spaces, meaning, and gesture in signed languages. *Cognitive Linguistics,* 15(2), 119–147.

Wilcox, S. (2004b). Hands and bodies, minds and souls: What can signed languages tell us about the origins of signs? In M. Alac & P. Violi (Eds.), *In the beginning: Origins of semiosis,* 137–167. Turnhout, Belgium: Brepols.

Wilcox, S., Shaffer, B., Jarque, M. J., Valenti, J. M. S. I., Pizzuto, E., & Rossini, P. (2000). *The emergence of grammar from word and gesture: A cross-linguistic study of modal verbs in three signed languages.* Paper presented at the seventh international conference on Theoretical Issues in Sign Language Research, Amsterdam, July 23–27.

Wilson, F. R. (1998). *The hand: How its use shapes the brain, language, and human culture.* New York: Pantheon Books.

Wylie, L., & Stafford, R. (1977) *Beaux gestes: A guide to French body talk.* Cambridge: Undergraduate Press.

Index